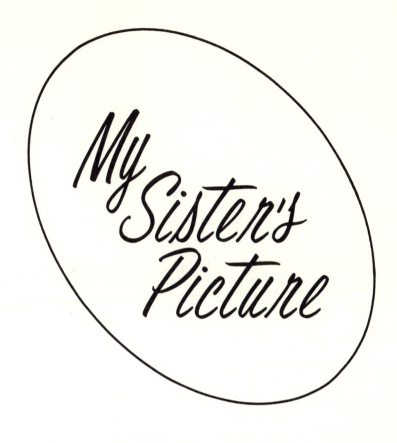

My Sister's Picture

Cathy Arden

SIMON AND SCHUSTER   NEW YORK

Published by Simon and Schuster
A Division of Simon & Schuster, Inc.
Simon & Schuster Building
Rockefeller Center
1230 Avenue of the Americas
New York, New York 10020
SIMON AND SCHUSTER and colophon are registered
trademarks of Simon & Schuster, Inc.
Designed by Helen L. Granger/Levavi & Levavi
Manufactured in the United States of America
10 9 8 7 6 5 4 3 2 1
Library of Congress Cataloging-in-Publication Data
Arden, Cathy.
    My sister's picture.

    1. Arden, Doren, d. 1981—Health.   2. Breast—
Cancer—Patients—United States—Biography.
I. Title.
RC280.B8A73   1986   362.1'9699449'00922 [B]   86-13119
ISBN: 0-671-50467-3

As a courtesy, the names of certain individuals in *My Sister's Picture* have been changed.

The author gratefully acknowledges the authors and publishers for use of the excerpts from the following:

C. S. Lewis, *A Grief Observed* (London: Faber and Faber Limited, © 1961 by C. S. Lewis).
Joni Mitchell, "Electricity," © 1972 Crazy Crow Music (BMI). Used by permission. All rights reserved.
Susan Sontag, *Illness as Metaphor* (New York: Random House, © 1977, 1978 by Susan Sontag).
Allen Toussaint, "Shoo-rah! Shoo-rah!" © 1973 Warner-Tamerlane Publishing Corp. & Marsaint Music, Inc. All rights reserved. Used by permission.

Acknowledgments

I am deeply grateful to Pat Golbitz, for her time and guidance throughout the entire process of this book, her creative vision, her soul that has touched these pages.

For their belief in the work, thanks to my editor at Simon & Schuster, Patricia Soliman, and my agent, Elaine Markson; and to Jane Low, in copyediting, for her patience and dedication.

Thanks also to C.M., for her invaluable contribution, to Dorien Ross, *amiga de mi alma*, to Trebor, for the songs.

A special thank you to my mother, for her faith in me and her support, and to George, for his understanding and expertise.
And to Rod, for his courage, his love, for reminding me what it is that survives.

FOR MY MOTHER
FOR MY FATHER

FOR ROD

You wonder how the man who comes to tune the piano
does it
so many strings

Where is the melody
and how fast?

My mother's hands are as unmysterious
to me as my own
further than that
everything is mystery

The bones and veins
as if my sister's spirit moved into
her hands as she died

something to memorize.

Our hands on the piano. Playing Chopsticks. Playing Heart and Soul.

That is one of the pictures.

One fall day, during Doren's freshman year at Bryn Mawr, she told me she began running down a hill to her dorm when she heard her favorite song wafting faintly toward her from someone's radio. She had to hear it up close. She tripped and fell halfway down the hill. When Doren told me this story she laughed. "I fell on my face for 'Walk Away Renee,' " she said. Later, she sent me the words to that song written out in perfect script on loose-leaf paper.

That is another picture.

When Doren was three years old she informed our parents she had to have a baby sister. A year later I was born. Doren often reminded me I had her to thank for this. Was I supposed to feel grateful, needed, loved? I never quite knew, but I know I believed it was my sister's idea that I come into being. I came into the world, then, Doren's child.

Prologue

My sister and I were always told that we came from a long line of eccentrics. As we grew up we checked ourselves at various stages, looking for the telltale signs, wondering if we, too, were joining the eccentric ranks. The word held its mystery, of course, and when we inquired as to its meaning, we would be told a story about a relative, a story which had earned that particular grandparent, aunt, or cousin the eccentric label.

It was only later I discovered that the world presents itself in such a way as to require everyone to be eccentric at one time or another. The predicament of grief is like this. As C. S. Lewis notes in *A Grief Observed*, "An odd by-product of my loss is that I'm aware of being an embarrassment to everyone I meet. . . . Perhaps the bereaved ought to be isolated in special settlements like lepers." I don't think this idea would work, however. The truth is, the bereaved appear odd even to each other. Although my mother, my father, and I all suffer the loss of the same person, the manifestations of our separate grieving are strange and foreign to each other.

Grief is mostly a possessive companion. It is so demanding it rarely allows for recognition of anyone else's grief—even when it belongs to someone close to you. When one does become aware of the other's awkward maneuvering around loss, the awareness produces a kind of embarrassment, like painful shyness. This awkwardness, grief's eccentricities, reveals itself in my family's diverse reactions to my sister's picture.

When my sister died my parents immediately constructed arrangements of her photographs in their respective homes. The most concentrated display of Doren's face in my mother's house is in her bedroom, on the dresser. The dresser is by the door, so the photographs are impossible to miss on one's way out of the room. I was startled the first time I saw my mother pass by her dresser, pick up one of the framed photographs in both hands, and kiss it. Not cautiously, as one might kiss a sleeping child, but enthusiastically, a few successive, audible kisses, the sort that might cause a young child to giggle and squirm. In this case, although I was neither the young child nor the recipient, I was the one who squirmed. When I expressed my discomfort at my mother's unabashed, eccentric gesture, she was surprised by my astonishment. Her impulse was as natural to her as the same impulse was when Doren was alive. She had always been affectionate toward her daughters, so why curb her instinctive gestures now? When someone you love dies, it is impossible to stop sending love out, impossible to believe it is no longer being received.

The focal point for the pictures in my father's home is on his desk. I have seen him lean back in his desk chair and then begin to rock the chair slightly as he looks at the photographs, his hand over his mouth as if to stop any sound from escaping. Prominent in his collection are photographs of Doren when she was a young teenager. The more recent ones, as a grown woman, taken just previous to her becoming ill, are in remotely visible areas of his living room. In contrast, my mother has the more recent pictures in her most prominent display. It has been difficult, she says, to fend off the images of Doren ill. The recent photographs help to remind her, she says, of her daughter healthy. My father needs to go even further back, envisioning a time as distant as possible from the present reality, a time more innocent of death.

I, on the other hand, have had photographs of my sister hidden away in various drawers and dark corners of my house. Two years after her death, I did not feel courageous enough to bring them out. I would not see them unless a specific choice to do so was made. I was under the impression that if these pictures were always in full view, my sister's image would be in danger of receding—much like a painting on the wall seen every day, growing less and less noticeable with time.

There was one, however, that found its way between the blank pages at the end of my appointment book. This way it would appear in view casually and by accident, and every few days I would catch a brief glimpse of Doren. It is a picture of her sitting on the grass at her favorite place, a farm in Virginia, the home of her closest friend, Candice—the place where now her ashes are buried. The shock of seeing her so alive became less overwhelming. I began to recognize again her tentative smile, the soft tilt of her head, the dark waves of her hair. A quiet, slow comfort crept in.

Now, as I write, I look up at the wall in front of me and Doren is in full view. I have brought the pictures out of hiding. For three years grief for my sister replaced her presence in my life. Now that the image of Doren is before me every day, she is not receding at all. I don't feel there is that danger anymore. I am allowing my sister re-entry.

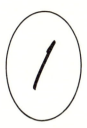

I am three or four years old, in the small room with the curtains that rain green cats and dogs. It's two in the afternoon and I'm waking up from my nap. The sun is seeping in through the openings in the curtains and making a skinny stream of light on the fuzzy emerald carpeting. There are voices below my window on the pink patio. The smell is sweet and warm and travels through my body, making me giggle. I giggle louder so Mommy will hear. She comes in and dresses me in my bathing suit with the little purple pussycats on it that ties around my neck and sometimes hurts. I don't mind, though, because I love purple pussycats. I can't wait to go outside on the patio, to be with Mommy, Daddy, and Doren, and sit in my green square wading pool with a yellow seat in every corner. (I hope there are no leaves floating in the pool.)

It is a hot summer morning in July. Sunday, and everyone is feeling happy. It's a beach day. My mother, father, sister, and I are all in the kitchen pitching in. There are egg-salad sandwiches being made on soft white bread with a few pieces of lettuce. The sandwiches are wrapped in wax paper. Tangerines are put in the powder-blue Styrofoam cooler. And green seedless grapes. Oreos, too. My father carries everything out to the car to put in the trunk. The large green, red, blue, and yellow striped beach umbrella is already in there. It stays in the trunk all summer long. He puts in the cooler with the old, frayed, quilted summer blanket. There are towels you can hide your whole body in, especially if you are five years old.

There was always something magical about a beach day. It was when my family was most peaceful. Doren and I would climb into the back seat of the blue Pontiac. On the way to Jones Beach, we counted how many things we saw out the window that began with the letter A, then B, then C. I would dare Doren to wave at the people in the car in back of us. We asked each other questions like: If I gave you a million dollars, would you lick the street even if you knew you'd get very sick afterwards? If I gave you a million dollars, would you give me your favorite stuffed animal to keep forever? If I looked like this (we would, alternately, put one finger on the tips of our noses, lift our noses up so that we looked like pigs), would you still love me? To this question Doren would always say "Yes" automatically. I would always say "No." Doren would laugh and say, "Oh, come on!" and she'd ask me over and over again, holding the tip of her nose up, waiting for me to say "Yes." "Well, *I* would love you no matter *what*," she'd proclaim, finally giving up.

My father would watch us in the rearview mirror, exclaim "Girls!" every once in a while. This would encourage us to come up with more and more outrageous questions. Mother would shift in her seat to look at us, concerned that our joking might turn into a fight. But in the car going to Jones Beach it never did. In the car going to Jones Beach there was a lot of laughing in the front seat and in the back seat.

My father wore his beige cotton shorts and no shirt. He'd unload the trunk when we arrived and dole out things to carry. Doren and I carried our pails and shovels. Mother carried the blanket. Father carried the umbrella and the cooler. And then we'd have to walk a long way over what seemed like miles of beach to find an uncrowded spot near the water. I looked at my father's bare feet a lot, amazed at how large they were. I'd put my foot up to his foot to compare, and tease him.

The sand. I hated it. I loved being with my family on beach days, but I hated the sand. I was constantly brushing myself off. I hated, too, the crunch of sand in the egg-salad sandwiches and the sting on my shoulders by the afternoon. I liked the colors of my pail and shovel, bright red and bright yellow, more than I liked to play with them. What I liked to do most was watch my father swim in the ocean. I was afraid of the ocean. The seaweed stuck to my feet and got in between my toes, and the waves were too powerful and out of control. Out of my control.

My father loved the ocean. I never saw him so happy and cheerful as he was on those beach days. He would always ask Doren and me to come with him into the water. Doren would always go, and I'd watch him lift her above the waves. My mother would encourage me to go, too, she'd say my father would protect me, I'd tell her I was afraid he'd drop me, and she'd say softly and firmly that he would never, ever do that. Doren would come back to the blanket after a short while, grinning madly, and after Mother helped her dry off, she'd squint into the sun, trying to make out which dot on the waves was my father. When he returned he'd report to me that there was no seaweed today, that the water was very calm, and why didn't I come in with him the next time. Maybe, I'd say. Just maybe.

Every once in a while I did, toward the end of the afternoon, close to leaving. It would be my last chance, his last swim. He'd take my hand as soon as we left the blanket. When we reached the water I'd let it skim my toes and would think about running back up to my mother and sister, to safety. Mother and Doren would wave, and their wave would turn into gestures urging me to go into the water. I'd wait on the shore for a while as my father dove into a wave. He would come back wet and his hand around mine would be cold. I promise, he'd say, to hold you the entire time and not let you go under a wave. I'd inch forward with him, screaming but still moving forward. He would pick me up in his arms and carry me into that frightening ocean.

And my father was true to his word. He lifted me above the waves, never loosening his grip around my waist. I would shriek and he would laugh. After a few minutes, in spite of my fear and discomfort, and the not very familiar feeling of being in my father's arms, I would start to laugh too. I was happy there with him. I'd look over my shoulder at Mother and Doren waving like crazy, and applauding, as I trusted my father to protect me from danger and keep me aloft.

Even though my mother was not a swimmer, she would join my father at the water too. They'd stand on the shore together, their backs to Doren and me wrapped in towels on the blanket, and it seemed those moments were the only glimpses I had of my parents' intimacy. The unity I experienced in my family on beach days. It was a unity I searched for at home, but there it seemed to slip away like the slow and quiet water receding from the shore, turning into a crashing wave again.

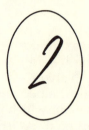

I am living in a makeshift home with the piano from
my childhood and my sister's desk. I have lived here,
alone, for ten years. I left for nine months and I have
recently returned. I hadn't planned on nine months. I
hadn't planned on returning. I hadn't planned on continuing to live in a makeshift house. I hadn't planned
on my sister's desk. My desk, the one I had built a
number of years ago that is no longer suitable by itself,
is now joined with my sister's desk. The two, together, form an "L." Her desk has drawers, mine does
not. But mine is wider, I can slide my typewriter to the
back when not in use and have room for writing by
hand. I have painted my desk white to match my sister's desk. The upside-down "L" is uniform.

A Salvation Army truck arrives this week to pick up
many boxes I have packed after having been away for
nine months. If I could do without all these things for
that long, I can do without them forever. In one of
those boxes is a small burgundy satin drawstring
pouch that Doren bought me for dancing at Studio 54.
Perhaps I had used it once, draped across my body,
the bag bouncing on my hip which heaved to Donna
Summer's "Last Dance." Perhaps that was another
drawstring bag. Perhaps I never used the burgundy
pouch at all. It took a week before I made the decision
to give this gift from Doren away.

I don't know what to cherish anymore. The piano my
sister and I played together? The desk my sister used for her
writing? What stays with me, what gets thrown out? Who performed the abracadabra that suddenly transformed Doren's belongings into mine? When we were children it was all I could
do to keep my hands off anything that was hers. Whatever
belonged to Doren I automatically loved, hoped would soon be
mine, and cherished whether it ended up in my room or not.
And still there are cartons stuffed into the highest closet

shelves in my mother's house. Cartons we brought to Doren's apartment and packed with all her things, dazed, the day after she died. I have been going through those cartons for over three years now. Slowly, very slowly, they have lessened in number. Now I look around at what has turned into a make-shift home. A home that is not altogether mine. But a home which includes my sister.

What can I let go of, what do I need to keep with me? Doren becomes translated so often into objects. Sometimes I am inclined to hold on to those objects for dear life. For Doren's dear life. Sometimes I am inclined to destroy them.

For the first twelve years of my life, and for the first sixteen years of Doren's, we lived in a corner house on a dead-end street in a suburban town called Merrick. As far as Doren was concerned, the town's only attribute was that it was only an hour's drive, or train ride, away from New York City. New York City was a place Doren felt she had to live in as soon as possible. It was a place I would have despised altogether were it not for Leonard Bernstein and the New York Philharmonic Orchestra, which my parents sometimes took me to hear. When Doren was twelve and I was eight, we were sometimes left to ourselves for an evening while our parents went off to "the city." Doren was my favorite baby-sitter.

In back of the house was a canal, a place where teenagers would often park their cars and "neck," as my parents described it. Sometimes, when Doren and I were by ourselves, we'd peek out my bedroom window, which afforded a full view of the canal, and we'd squint, trying to discern figures and movement in cars. Pressed up against the glass, squinting and giggling, was more fun for me not because of what I imagined to be going on under those convertible tops, but because I was squinting and giggling with my sister and feeling silly instead of afraid.

On those long nights, waiting for our parents to return, I needed distraction. And Doren obliged. We obediently took on our respective roles: Cathy is terrified; Doren comforts Cathy. As far as I knew, Doren was never afraid. Not of lightning, not of moonless nights, not of ghosts, not of witches. My sister would stave off anything wicked, for my sake. I would curl up into my sister's body as we watched television on our parents' queen-size bed. In this way I could brave the scary pictures. Before Dorothy's house hit the ground in *The Wizard of Oz*, before the red-and-white-striped stockings appeared on the screen, Doren would place her full hand over my eyes as I squirmed and screeched. She'd place her hands over my ears right before the wicked witch in the black cape cackled and I would hum a camp song as she did this to help block out the eerie sound. If a storm passed over the house and lightning brightened my room, Doren would sit at the end of my bed, holding my feet tightly, affording me ground where I thought there was none. When a policeman came to our house early one evening asking questions because someone had fished up a dead baby in a tin toolbox out of the canal, Doren showed no fear. As I turned ashen, developing a picture of this baby and this tin box that would stay with me forever, Doren put one arm around my shoulders and said calmly, "I'm sorry, Officer, but our parents aren't home right now and my sister and I don't know anything about this. Can you please come back another time when our parents are here?"

In later years, when my fears of witches and lightning and other unknown things that seemed to come at me from the sky receded, Doren's job as distracter held firm. One weekend, when we were both in our twenties, we were together at my mother's country house. I was distressed over a relationship with a man that had gone awry. Nothing seemed to alleviate my feelings of hopelessness and I remember a frantic, desperate look creeping over my sister's face as she tried to figure out a way to distract me from despair. She invented games, word games on paper, told me bits of gossip that ordinarily would have made me laugh. If she saw my attention start to wane, that faraway look come into my eyes, she'd move quickly on to something else. The pitch of her voice began to rise in her fervent attempt to keep me from tears.

She devised a solution. "I'll give you a pedicure! I'll fix your toes!" My toes, I had always felt, were crooked and ugly and beyond repair. I was ashamed of wearing open-toed sandals in the summer or of baring my feet on any occasion. Now Doren intended to rid me of this lifetime insecurity. My sister was suddenly on the floor at my feet, small tools and a bottle of red nail polish beside her. When the operation was complete I lifted my feet out in front of me to examine them. These feet I had always loathed looked feminine, they looked the way I imagined female feet were supposed to look. And although my friends do not think of me as the pedicure type, I have continued Doren's tradition of painting my toes, explaining to those who are puzzled, "But, listen, you don't understand, this has to do with my sister. . . ."

My entering the world as Doren's child left Doren little time to be a child herself. She took on the attributes of an adult before most people's time, acting as friend to our mother, who was distressed in a troubled marriage, and as protector to her younger sister, who was distressed in a troubled home.

_____

Oh what a dream I had last night! Cathy and I were alone and we heard noises so we went down to the kitchen to call the police. The wire of the phone was cut and I really got scared. I ran next door to the Rosses, pulled out their kitchen phone, and plugged it in our socket. I went down the stairs to the basement and closed the door. "Operator, I want the police."

"One moment please."

"Operator, there are some men who are going to break in here in a minute. I want the police at 2787 Bay Drive, Merrick."

"One moment please."

"Damn it," I screamed, "get the police. 2787 Bay Drive, Merrick."

Just then Cathy opened the door. She was white. "Doren, some men are breaking in." "Oh God." Just then there were 2 or 3 men in the kitchen. One took Cathy, one took me. When I got outside I couldn't see Cathy but Father was there and I could see that he was the ringleader. "For God's sake, what are you doing?" I screamed. "Do anything to me but do you realize Cathy will stutter for the rest of her life? What did you do with her? Oh I *despise* you." "Look," he said. "I'm not stealing anything. Whatever I take from this house is *mine,* do you understand?" He was screaming and he looked like a beast. Police cars were coming and a whole crowd of people were milling around. "Whatever happens, no matter *what* happens, I will *never* forgive you for this! Never!" Just then Mother came. "That's right," she said, "you *know* she won't change her mind."

And Daddyo woke me up.

_____

If Doren was the protector and I was the fearful child, I tipped the balance when it came to physical strength. My physical power and Doren's physical weakness was another configuration we relished. For two summers we were together at the same all-girls summer camp, Trebor, in Maine. My favorite activity was to play tetherball with my sister. I'd pull her down to the landsports field, she acting as if she were reluctant to go but laughing all the way. How many times did I wrap the ball around the pole before she decided to give in? She'd try, though. She'd keep the game going, the inside of her wrist where she'd pound the ball would turn red, she'd shriek with excitement when it looked as if the ball was going to elude my fist, she'd brush away stray hairs sticking to her damp face and tuck them back under her white pixie band, and at some point after I had triumphed more than once, she'd say, "I give up," and she'd smile. Always she would agree to come down to the landsports field to play tetherball with me, knowing this was the place I was likely to win and she was likely to lose. "I don't know why I keep doing this," she'd say, walking arm in arm with me away from the landsports field, the tetherball still knocking gently against the pole behind us.

Doren wanted me to feel strong. I was a fearful child and she felt I needed her support and strength in a home where perhaps I was not getting enough of either. She had wanted me to be born in the first place, now she'd have to rescue me from whatever was to go wrong. As far as my sister was concerned, this was her responsibility. It was one she would never relinquish until the last years of her life when the battle she had to fight was no longer mine, or my mother's, or my father's, but hers alone.

Not one of my visitors this evening asked me if I felt afraid. Most people in fact advised me that there is absolutely no reason to be afraid. Everything is going to be fine, my family and friends inform me. No need to worry. Do *not* worry. We forbid you to worry.

Of course, I am worried, but not to the degree that I myself might have anticipated. There is no reality to this experience yet. I know I am here. I know I will undergo surgery tomorrow morning. Despite the odds being overwhelmingly in my favor, I also know that I wouldn't be here at all if there were no chance that something is terribly wrong. Nevertheless, I still feel like a strong young woman . . . well young woman. The mind may have weighed and understood the implications of this experience, but the soul has certainly not caught up with it yet.

I am still working on a more elementary piece of information: I have a lump in my left breast.

My breast. My lump.

Doren might be sick.
But Doren has no right.
Danny will not like sick Doren.
Jack will not like sick Doren.
Neither will Candice.
Nobody will.

Doren may not be diseased.
Doren had better not.

_____

When we were children I wanted Doren's courage as much as I wanted the purple canopy over her bed. If I stayed as physically close to her as possible, and as frequently as possible, at least I would reap the benefits of her courage if not take it on as my own. Snuggling in the canopied bed with her, my head fitting just under her arm, was the best shield I could have hoped for. We were allies; playing tent under quilted blankets on Sunday mornings, the smell of Matzoe Brie still in the air, hiding out from having to wash and dry the dishes, writing duets and then performing them for our parents. One of these songs in particular stayed with us into adulthood and one or the other of us would sing it over the phone on occasion to lift the spirits of whichever one of us was down at the time. "You're my bratty-pie, oohooohoooohoooh, when you kick me in the head/You're my bratty-pie, oohooohoooohoooh, when you knock me off the bed/I love you but do you love me/Oh I guess I'll never see/'Cause you're my bratty-pie/I wish you'd leave me alone, oohooohoooohoooh, my bratty-pie/And never ever come home, oohooohoooohoooh, sweet bratty-pie/I love you but do you love me/Oh I guess I'll never see/'Cause you're my bratty-pie. . . ."

With Doren I was comforted, I was safe. What I wasn't aware of was that she had a life that didn't include me, even when we were children. As long as I could count on my sister to be there for me when I needed her, the fact that she had experiences at school and with friends that didn't include me was, for a while, irrelevant.

_____

Today I went up thinking about the very distant past—winning contests as a lindy "artiste," for example—flashes that were followed by a recitation of all my elementary school teachers. First Grade—the white-haired, severe but decent Mrs. Allen. Second Grade—the young and sexy Miss Siegel, who made every story my favorite story (e.g., _My Father's Dragon_) and who taught me how to write script, and who used to tease fat Jerry Levine who ate too many doughnuts and said "liberry." . . . Jerry Levine was my first bad "heterosexual" trip. The first bottle I ever spun pointed at him. Perhaps that is the precise point at which I acquired my distaste for sexual games.

To continue—Third Grade—Mrs. Berg, the vicious battle-ax

who tied Barry Sands to his chair one day and stuffed him in a wastebasket another day and dragged me once across the room by my ponytail because I was committing the cardinal sin: talking. And who used to give a speech every day at five minutes to three which went something like, "Don't you children dare tell your parents what went on here today, because if any one of you should tell, I will find out which one it is and I will make that person very sorry. Very, very sorry."

And all of us three-foot-tall people cowering every time that five-foot-square old lady shoved her metal chair back from her desk. . . .

And the fact that it was me—three-foot Doren, ponytailed and spitcurled (one Betty Boop curl curved inward at the right temple) who finally broke, under the persistent interrogation of Mother (of course) and told all, and precipitated a flood of phone calls emanating from my house to mothers, fathers, Mr. Dorfman (the principal), etc., which in the end precipitated exactly nothing. Mrs. Berg had tenure and she was not fired until a few years later when she beat up on one little boy just once too often.

I remember wondering if it was being fat that made her so mean, or being old or having varicose veins. And I think I usually concluded that it must be the varicose veins, because they were exceedingly horrible.

And Fourth Grade—Mr. Walters, my first male teacher and my first real fan (barring my two parents and Cathy-as-a-child). Man did he love me. Everything I did was wonderful to him. He didn't have to say anything! When I answered a question in class he just beamed at me in a way that said, "It's kids like you, Doren, that make my job a gas."

I was teacher's pet that year. I loved it.

Even when it came time to do our class play, and in the democratic tradition of our class we cast by balloting, and Lynn Schwartz and I got tie votes three times in a row, and Mr. Walters put both of our names in a hat and drew one, and it was my name, and everyone who had voted for Lynn cried Foul Play and really, I wasn't sure myself if he had actually picked my name or had even written Lynn's name on either slip, because the minute he looked at the slip he tore up both slips into very small pieces and threw them in the garbage.

I can see myself climbing the steps into a big yellow bus that afternoon, and hearing the sound of jeers from behind me—the voices of some of Lynn's admirers (they liked her only because she had "real" breasts)—Lynn's admirers yelling, "You didn't win it fair, Doren. You didn't win it fair."

And I remember thinking as I climbed the last step into the bus,

"Wait until you get home to smile, Doren. Don't smile now. Don't let them see that you don't care how you won. Don't let them know you're glad you won, fair or not."

The part was in a play about mothers (because it was presented around Mother's Day) and my first line, the opening line of the play, was "Work, work, work, will there never be an end to it? It's just one thing after another just as fast as I can fly."

And I had on a pale blue "duster" over my costume for Act II, and I ran all over the set like a grounded, speeding Peter Pan, dusting everything in sight.

Another flash on that year—Walters insisted that the class be run like a democracy. On the first day of school he gave us a long lecture about how things would be in our mini-democracy. What it boiled down to was that we voted on things all the time—at least 5 times a day for small decisions; weekly decisions like who would clean the erasers, take out the garbage, give out tests, etc.; and monthly on who would be class president, vice president, and secretary. (When I tried to pull a Franklin Roosevelt, the class rebelled and made a law that forbade more than two consecutive terms as president. Later when I ran again, they ruled a limit of two terms, period.)

In keeping with the democracy, Walters made it possible for everyone in the class to succeed at something. There were at least twenty categories, and when he awarded prizes at the end of the year for individual categories, combinations, and all-around wonderfulness, everyone got at least one prize.

Guess who hit the jackpot that June, though? Guess who went home with one toppling armload of prizes and presents? (I've just slipped a little gold star out of the drawer of my desk, licked it, and pasted it in the center of my forehead. As a hint.)

And Fifth Grade—Mrs. McNeil, who called us "folks," which I didn't like. And who wore dark suede shoes with the big toe hanging out, which I didn't like. And whose breasts were very big and sagged down to her waist, which I also didn't like.

And Sixth Grade—Mr. Cadden, a young and sort of plump but sexy man. . . . I remember how excited we all got when we heard that his wife (who we never did meet) was going to have a baby. The vibrations were fun, but different, and kind of scary, and how we didn't even know enough to call it sexual excitement, didn't know yet that each of us was working out an intricate fantasy about Mr. Cadden in our minds, and that the baby meant all sorts of things to just about every person in the classroom.

That was the year that the "social life" went too far and starting in September the only truly important after-school topic of discussion was who was going to take who to the sixth-grade prom at the end of the year. Invitations began right away and, after that, breakups, and new invitations and more breakups. And the hostilities got so out of hand that one afternoon Mr. Cadden made about ten of us stay after school and discuss the whole thing and warned us that the fucking (he didn't use the word "fucking," but I seem to remember that he used some obscenity here that shocked us a lot, probably just "damn") that the fucking dance wasn't worth what we were making it be worth.

And how, sometime before the spring, it became acceptable— in the in-group—to fear and hate me. Even though I was pretty (not too tall, complete with "real" breasts), it became the thing not to like a girl who did so well in school and who in fact was the best student in the class and got 100's and 100-pluses all the time, and how by the time the prom came, I ended up going with someone who was not in the in-group, and who was more than a foot shorter than me. His name was Don.

The sadness of that year precipitated a great deal of crying and breast-beating under the theme of "I'm not popular anymore. I want to be popular but I'm not. I want to die."

Sitting on the toilet in Mother's bathroom one late weekday afternoon, I understood suicide for the first time, on (from what I can recall) a quite legitimate level, and how at that moment Mother picked up on a message that would plague me for many years and probably will plague me forever: Don't worry, darling. Someday you will meet a man who will love you for what you are and you will be so happy that you are who you are that it will make up for this time. It will be the greatest happiness in the world. (I wonder now what man she was thinking of then, or if she was only reciting a credo which had failed for her, but which she desperately hoped would work for her daughter.)

This was the other side of the argument I had heard from age three: Darling, I want you to know that I consider it a mistake that I married so early in life, and that I quit college, and I don't want you to make the same mistake. And I want you to know that it's all right with me if you have affairs. I don't think you should get married just because someone tells you it isn't right to have affairs, and I will support you in your decision, if you should decide not to listen to "what people say."

Mother says now that she would never have talked like that to a three-year-old. All I know is I remember that particular lecture as far back as early childhood, before Cathy was born. And that I was too ashamed to tell her that I didn't know what she meant by "affairs." It was not in my limited childhood vocabulary. Knowing Mother from the vantage point of the present, I would guess that she theorized that it "couldn't hurt" to tell me that message even if I was still too small to understand, because it would sink in somehow, if repeated often enough. And I think she was right, though the only part of it that worked was the don't-quit-college part. I hated college, but felt driven to finish mostly because I didn't want to let her down in such an enormous and devastating way. After being warned all my life, that would be too much.

The first time Doren began to withdraw from me is vivid. I was at least eight years old. I had always been able to assume that whenever I needed Doren, wanted Doren, she would make herself available to me. She and her best friend, Vivien, were going to a Saturday afternoon movie and, as always, I assumed I was going with them. Doren turned around to me (I was trailing behind her toward the front door) and said something clear and simple like, "No, Cathy." It was the first "No" I can recall that so totally baffled me. My sister, who had never said that word to me before, had in an instant altered the terms of our relationship. That "No" was instituting her right to be a person apart from me. That "No" was as unfamiliar to Doren as it was to me, and from that point forward she would never feel comfortable using it with me. On many occasions she would not say "No" when she would have preferred to. Resentments began to grow out of those moments of acquiescence. And my resentment grew when she would not acquiesce, when I experienced a separation I was not ready for.

The large resentment surfaced much later, when we were adults. It occurred after a period of many months in which I had silenced our relationship. Doren had already been treated for breast cancer, had had a lumpectomy, and was, we all thought, fine. This is when I stopped speaking to her. At the time I did not connect those two events—her cancer, my silence. There was something I thought I was angry at her about, something important enough to call a halt to any semblance of communication between us. I don't remember what I thought to be the cause of this anger. I surely did not know then that I was in a rage at my sister for forcing me into a new world, one in which I had to imagine the unimaginable—living without her. By severing ties for a number of months, was I instituting a trial run?

But the first time I felt alone and unprotected was on that Saturday afternoon when Doren walked out the front door with her friend Vivien, and without me. How was I going to brave the world without my one trusted ally? Along with a deep and vast loneliness, another feeling moved into that dark place. I felt betrayed.

Once this first separation began its course, I started noticing things I had never been aware of before. Because I wasn't by Doren's side every minute, I began seeing new things from a distance. Every day, after Doren came home from school in the late afternoon, I would hear repeated thuds against the wall separating our bedrooms. I would put my ear to my side of the wall trying to identify these strange sounds. What I could hear pressed up against the wall was something else that was familiar although I hadn't heard it very often. It was the sound of my sister crying. I had no idea what she was crying about, or what the thuds were, but for the sadness that began to spread through my body, I might as well have been crying for her. She may have begun to separate from me, but my connection to her could not be severed.

One day, after the thuds and the crying had stopped, and I was discreetly walking by Doren's closed bedroom door, she opened it suddenly and I smiled at her so she wouldn't know of my distress. She said quietly, "Do you want to see something?" I nodded and walked over the threshold I was amazed was not forbidden me. "This is what I do every day when I come home from school," Doren said, picking a rather battered apple up off the purple carpet. "I throw apples against the wall, like this—" And she gave me a demonstration. There was a spot on the wall from the juice of apples, and it served as Doren's bull's-eye. She asked me if I wanted to try throwing one myself. I declined her offer. This was my first glimpse of Doren's unhappiness. I felt helpless, ineffectual. I didn't ask questions. I didn't take my eyes off the bruised apple and the bruised wall.

How to prevent insanity at home:

1. Leave the room when the conversation becomes unnerving, or better yet, see that dangerous topics—e.g., school—are avoided.

2. When Mother is on the phone try to close your ears and concentrate hard on something else.

3. When you hate your family, think that they'll be dead someday and you'll be punishing yourself for hating them now.

4. When you start to cry, concentrate on an object. Look at it and just keep saying its name in your head until it means nothing and your mind is empty . . . doorknob, doorknob, doorknob, doorknob, etc.

5. If you're really angry, pour all your strength into some concentrated physical act. Biting a pen or a pencil, digging your fingernails into your palms until you feel weak, or throwing some apples against your bedroom wall. (Four are enough if you re-use each one until it's squashed.)

6. If nothing helps—even writing 300 times "Goddamn . . ." —see if you can kill yourself yet. Fill the sink with water. If you come up for air when you can't breathe, then things aren't so bad. . . .

What difference am I to the world? Even to my "friends" and family? (P.S. I've ruined my sister and she hates me.)

————————

Had she brought me into her room to show me the apple so that I would become aware of her distress—and *do* something? Was she trying to initiate then a switching of roles and asking me in some way for protection? Did she want me to stop needing her? I wasn't easily weaned. Her guilt at saying "No" to me at all produced her fear that I was growing to hate her.

There were two potent dramas developing in our house. There was the drama between sisters and the drama between husband and wife. When the one between our mother and father became fierce, Doren and I would suspend our own and jump into theirs in an effort to somehow set things right. Of course this was a futile effort, but it didn't stop us from frequently getting in the middle.

It is impossible for a child of divorced parents to ever really know the deepest reasons that led to the divorce, and foolhardy to theorize about them. I know only the surface information—that my parents married very young (my mother had been in her late teens and my father not much older) and that they were passionately in love; as they matured, their differences emerged. The stress of maintaining an intimate relationship and raising children, and their concerns about financial matters, pressed in on them. My sister remembered our parents' early passion. I remember the passionate discord.

I feared my father's temper, his tendency to throw things in a fit of rage. When I heard his voice begin to rise behind my parents' bedroom door, and my mother's voice growing softer the louder his became, I'd rush into their room, see them in a standoff, my mother's face tear-drenched, my father's face a threatening red, and I'd throw myself against my mother, my back against her stomach, my arms outstretched to protect her. I imagined blows that never existed. I would scream at my father to leave her alone, he would scream for me to get out of the room, then Doren would come running in screaming at my father not to hurt me. When this scenario took place, my father, exasperated, would storm out of the room. Mother would attend to her two daughters, who were, by this time, in a frenzy. Long after Doren calmed down, I'd still be screaming after my father, using curse words I had learned from my friends.

Whatever natural separation might have occurred between Doren and me was thwarted by the fact that we were continually thrown together either to defend our mother, defend our parents' marriage, or to try to control situations that were never within our control. We were compelled to stick together. Separate, we were powerless.

There was just a terse little discussion in the next room. . . . Exit Daddyo to studio—SLAM. Miscellaneous comments—"Is this the way to restore a marriage?" (Father.) "You are *hostile*." (Mother.) Why don't they get divorced and get the hell over with it? A quick bomb would be a lucky break for this whole family.

I think my parents are going to be divorced this year. If it doesn't happen soon, it never will. Years ago I would have been hysterical, now I'm sitting calmly recording my thoughts without a trace of emotion. It really doesn't frighten me anymore.

When we heard our parents fighting it seemed there had been no specific catalyst. It wasn't clear just what was causing all the anger. Anger in our house was amorphous, it wasn't anything you could pin down and name. There was one time, however, that Doren and I got wind of what the yelling was all about. My father was working as a television filmmaker and public relations specialist in the medical and health fields. He wrote, directed, and produced the films and sometimes appeared on screen as well, as an interviewer or announcer. The upheaval, connected on a certain level with his work, was so significant that it was the first time a separation between our parents seemed imminent.

Although we had long been aware of my father's decidedly precarious ego, it nevertheless came as a shock to learn that he had actually undergone plastic surgery at forty.

The terrors of watching his nose hammered down to a blob of putty in preparation for the surgical magic that would transform him from a neurotic, aging Jewish boy into a confident, fine-nosed imitation of Tyrone Power were certainly nothing compared to the terrors unleashed by his wife when she learned of the act.

"Who was that on the telephone, Doren?" my mother asked as she diced the onions.

"It was Daddy," I said quietly, trying to figure out the best way to tell her what I had just discovered.

"Oh? Didn't he want to speak to me? Did he tell you when he's coming home?"

"He'll be home in a few hours."

"Really? Well, didn't he want me to pick him up at the airport?"

"He didn't take a plane."

"What? What do you mean? He's been at a public relations convention in Chicago for four days. How else would he get home?"

"Mommy, he didn't go to Chicago. . . ." My mother eyed me suspiciously, wondering, no doubt, if my father had finally cracked and admitted an adulterous affair to his eleven-year-old daughter. I continued calmly, little knowing that what I was about to tell her would be taken as hard as adultery, if not harder. "He's been at some hospital in Manhattan getting a nose job."

My mother blanched, then went red, then commenced rolling her eyes in an awesome combination of rage and helplessness.

"He wanted me to prepare you before he got home, in case you might be frightened by his bandages."

My mother said nothing for several minutes. Then she left her onions and went upstairs to her bedroom. Before she slammed the door, I heard her mutter, "Filthy bastard." Or maybe it was "Fucking bastard."

She was still upstairs when my father returned. My sister and I met him at the front door, anxious to see if he looked scarier than usual. He didn't look too bad—just a little gray around the eyes; the bandage across the bridge of his nose was modest, indeed.

"Why did you do it, Daddy?" I inquired.

"Well, Doren, I hope to be doing more television in the future, and the fact of the matter is, my old nose just didn't photograph well enough."

"It looked okay to me," ventured my sister bravely.

My father's agreeable tone vanished and he said tersely, "Well, it wasn't. . . . Where's your mother?"

"She's been upstairs ever since I told her."

"How did she take it? Could you tell?"

"She's not too happy about it."

My father shrugged, dropped his suitcase and jacket on the bench in the hall, and marched upstairs to the bedroom. His entrance provoked bloodcurdling screams.

The onions lay abandoned on the cutting board; there would be no home cooking tonight. My sister and I put some TV dinners in the oven, and by the time they were done, the battle seemed nowhere near its finale.

My sister and I involved ourselves totally in a discussion about who would get the chicken dinner and who the beef. It was easy for me to convince her that the beef was preferable because the chicken dinners were reported to contain a certain chemical harmful to growth.

As I sucked fried chicken off the last small bones, I tried to hear what was going on upstairs, but it was difficult owing to the distance and the language-obscuring volume of it all. I did hear my mother's voice ask repeatedly, "How COULD you?" and my father's voice boom more than once, "What I do with my nose is MY BUSINESS!"

We were just throwing the aluminum trays into the garbage when my father bolted down the stairs and into the kitchen.

"I'm leaving," he announced. "Your mother doesn't want me to live here anymore."

My sister took the news quite calmly, but I burst into tears. I flung myself at him. "Don't go, Daddy. We want you to stay, don't we?" I looked at my sister for support.

She said nothing.

"Well, *I* want you to stay. Please, please don't go. I need you!"

"I'm sorry," he said as he removed me from his suit like a loose thread. "I can't stay here, I have to go."

He returned to the front hall, put on his jacket, picked up his pre-packed suitcase, and reached for the front door.

He was halfway out the door when my sister appeared behind him, tugging at his pants leg.

He turned with considerable irritation.

"Would you give me a souvenir?"

"What?"

"A souvenir of you."

He grimaced, wrinkling the bandage on his nose, and walked out.

Despite the fact that my father did come home that night, and many nights after that, for my sister and me that day would always be the significant occasion when we started adjusting to the idea of fatherlessness.

Years ago I tended to recall only the personal trauma of that night, but in time my mother's response began to seem even more compelling. I became convinced it was the shock of betrayal—the sudden realization that my father wanted a new face regardless of her feelings about his old one—and the subsequent shock of losing influence over him to another (Vanity?) that unbalanced her so completely.

————————

During those early years in Merrick, when it was all I could do to keep up with the changing formations in the familial choreography, there was, on occasion, a visitor in our house. My maternal grandfather, who lived with my mother's sister in Wilmington, Delaware, would sometimes come and stay with us for extended periods of time. Everyone loved this man, whose name was Abraham. I boasted to my friends that my grandfather was Abraham Lincoln. I believed this until the disappointing day when I learned his last name was Waretnik.

I feared my grandfather. Or rather, I feared his age. I didn't understand why, when he smiled, I saw only raw, pink gums without teeth. Or why I had to give up *Romper Room* when I'd come home from school for lunch and have to watch my grandfather's favorite television personality, Arthur Godfrey. I would sit with him in front of the television, eating my sugared sour cream and bananas, while my grandfather would fill me in on the merits of Arthur Godfrey.

My sister was always folded into Grandfather's lap—a place coveted by her and one that was anything but revered by me.

————————

As solid as two drinking straws
my grandfather's legs
float above
crabbed feet
aflame even in cool sand.
My grandfather, a tourist in
boxer trunks
wide enough for two men;
inhabitant of papier-mâché skin
which, sunburned, appears
a partly rouged and melting
paste

is holding out his arms (a
characteristic

move). He wants to swing me
over the waves; he offers me
my favorite fun.

My grandfather knows.
He's the only one who's guessed
that I was born
too soon; that I suffer a
constant and a growing need
for the comfort of familial
flesh. Permitting me
always
to feast on his,
he has become my
wetnurse and my principal
childhood meal.

I am wishing (just before I run
to him) that this time I may
adhere to his soft,
hairless chest—
a toasted marshmallow
his permanent
kangaroo-child.

———————

I was jealous of Doren's relationship with Grandpa. Why couldn't I love him like she did? Why was it different for me? And if I could bring myself to love him, then perhaps I, too, could sit in his lap and be loved. I couldn't get past my aversion. It was as if he knew this and provoked me just for fun. Like the time he needed to use the bathroom, which I refused to vacate, regardless of his repeated requests. Later he took me by the hand downstairs to the kitchen, pointed out the window at a darkened spot on the pink patio where, he said, because of me, he had had to relieve himself. "Look what you made me do!" he scolded. I refused to believe what he was telling me, and I finally broke free and ran back upstairs. I knew he wasn't *really* angry, and my sister, mother, and father would laugh and reassure me when I told them "what happened with Grandpa," but I just could never reconcile myself to a man who was older than anyone else I had ever come into contact with. His presence in the house brought something unpleasant close to me. It brought the contemplation of death. And then it brought death itself.

I was seven years old when Grandfather died. My family, along with an entire neighborhood, slipped into grief. I knew my mother, sister, and father were crying by their red eyes— no one cried in front of me. I didn't understand this. It was not as if I had never seen the members of my family cry before. Grief, in my house, was being kept a secret.

Grandfather had become ill in Wilmington and, once in the hospital there, it was discovered he had had a heart attack. My mother immediately took off for Delaware. I don't recall whether or not my father went with her, but I was deposited at the home of my best friend. I didn't know where my sister was, nor did I have access to her. I was frightened and home-sick to the point of nausea. I pretended to be just fine. I kept my feelings to myself, and I had no idea why they existed at all. It was years later that I found out Doren had been shipped off to the home of her best friend as well. In the midst of turmoil, I did not seem to have this information. I know that during the time my mother and father were away, I did not speak to my sister.

My mother returned to Merrick before her father died, she brought me home, and then the phone call came giving her the news of his death. She dropped the receiver and fled to her bedroom. I sat in the kitchen, watching the dangling receiver bounce off the wall, and I was then taken back to my friend's house. I was separate from my family once again. I cried quietly, in my pillow at night or behind a locked bathroom door. I took the cue from the rest of my family that no one should be witness to this emotion, this grief. For the first time I felt physically unsafe, and I was without my sister.

My mother's desire was to protect me. I was too young, too vulnerable, she thought, to be exposed to death. By keeping me from an acknowledgment of grief, I suppose she felt she was keeping me from death. When she returned from the funeral the family was back together again under one roof. But it was a gloomy family. Out of desperation, I gave myself a job. Court jester. I made it my business to cheer everyone up, to entertain, and produce laughter. I had a mission, I had purpose. I found my place. It was the only way I could include myself and feel active within the mystery of grief.

It worked. My family began to depend on me to alleviate their darkness. I felt connected, in control, needed. As I danced and sang and comforted the grown-ups, my own fear, held in abeyance, went unnoticed. This habit took root and grew up with me. It kept me only partially turned toward the world as more and more I moved toward solitude. Surely, I thought, I would be rejected if I stopped the humor and the song and the dance and stood in the middle of everything, just me and my nasty grief.

The world was subtly becoming a place where people were moving away from me. The first person I blamed was my sister. She was trying so hard to claim independence, but in doing so she would have to leave me behind.

"Please come out, now. I give up, I can't find you. Do you hear me? Come back! Please, I said I give up!"

The only sound is the summer wind moving through the leaves on the old maple tree in the front yard. I run around the whole outside of the house, searching under bushes, up in trees, in the porch, behind the swings, down those big holes the trees in back are standing in, and by the canal. I still can't find my sister. Doren always wants to play hide and seek. "Maybe *this* time you'll find me," she says. But I never can and she never comes when I call. I stand in front of the garage, tasting the liverwurst from lunch behind my nose, waiting for Doren to come around the corner. Suddenly, like magic, she's standing next to me, leaning against the garage door. "It was the wind," Doren says, "the wind took me away again."

She says this time it carried her away while I was still counting. "Yes, yes, that gust of wind when you were up to ten." She flew above the maple tree, across the canal, and up to the palace in the sky. There is always a feast waiting for Doren up there, laid out on the purple rug: grapes (without seeds), soft ice cream, bitter-sweet chocolate, raisin bread and apple cider.

Doren says, "The wind wants me to stay and live there, but he always takes me back when I want to go home."

"No, it's not true. The wind doesn't take you." (The lump in my throat makes my voice shake.) But I can never find her.

"Why won't he take *me*? Prove that it's true."

"He only likes *me*," Doren says. "No one else can ever come."

She walks away taking a Hershey Kiss from her pocket. I follow her.

"Tell me what it's like to fly with the wind."

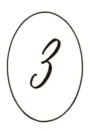

I am twelve years old, sitting on the bare wood floor in a dark room that is longer than it is wide. It is the first night in our new home in New York City. I am crying. Doren is sitting on the floor next to me, holding my hand, stroking my head, encourgaging me to sing camp songs with her. ". . . Peace I ask of thee, oh river, peace, peace, peace. . . .When I learn to live serenely, cares will cease. . . . From the hills I gather courage, visions of the day to be. . . . Strength to lead and faith to follow, all are given unto me. . . ." Her hand is softer than anything I have ever touched. Her face is radiant in the light shining in from the hallway. No one, I think, is more beautiful. I wish I had her dark wavy hair. I wish I looked like her. I wish I was not so unhappy.

The nurse has come into the hospital room to give my sister another shot for pain. I am trying to encourage Doren to sing a camp song with me, to distract her from agony. I am not sure she knows who I am now, but sometimes she remembers the words to a particular song—"Peace I ask of thee, oh river, peace, peace, peace. . . ." After the nurse leaves I adjust the silk scarf on Doren's bald head. Even now, she is beautiful. Doren stirs into consciousness for a few moments —"Remember," she keeps saying to me, over and over again. She reaches out with her hand that is black and blue and cold and touches my face and says, "Remember . . . remember . . . it's nice to remember . . . I remember you, I remember you. . . ." She feels my eyes, my cheeks, touches my hair, puts her hand on my head. "I remember everything, remember everything . . . it's nice . . . it's nice to remember everything . . . I remember you. . . ." This time I let her see me cry. She keeps her hand on my wet face. I say, "I remember everything, I remember you." Her eyes close, then suddenly she frowns and winces, puts her hand to her own face, a gesture I have learned means she is in pain. But she says, "Oh, I just remembered . . . it reminded me . . . I remember . . . I remember . . ." She is crying. "Doren." My sister opens her eyes, looks straight at me. "I love you," I say. "I love you, too," she says. And her eyes close again.

I did not agree with the family consensus that it was time for us to pack up and leave Merrick and move into The City. At twelve years of age I had not yet begun to feel oppressed by the confines of suburbia. Doren apparently had felt this oppression for quite a while and at sixteen the move to New York City was way overdue as far as she was concerned. Our parents were both working in Manhattan; Mother had begun to work in the publicity department at a publishing firm and my father's filmmaking work was based in New York. Doren, for six months before we moved, was commuting every day as well, to a private school in New York. She had managed to convince my mother, who then managed to convince my father, that she would not survive if she were to begin her junior year of high school in the Merrick public school system. Doren was what everyone called "highly motivated . . . gifted," and apparently needed no other pressure to work than the exorbitant amount of pressure she put on herself. As Doren became an adolescent, she felt a growing isolation from her classmates and friends. As hard as she sometimes tried, she just couldn't maneuver her personality to fit in. But Doren did not want to feel like a misplaced citizen. She was compelled to associate herself with the in-crowd.

I was just in the girls' room with the little hoods. They despise me I know and I usually just don't say anything but next time I will. The girl hoods call me Mona Lisa and the boy hoods call me Smiley. I turned around and as I looked around the room three girls were all staring at me with *that look*. . . .

I measure school relationships by "Do you say hello in the halls?" or "Would you ask him (her) for a ride home?" Well, I'm always helloing now and last Saturday night I went home with Laura Kamen, Linda Grey, Floyd Kayne, Rick March, and Barbara Schwartz—all highly respected seniors, especially Floyd, Rick, and Linda,—*brains*—but let me qualify. . . .

Floyd—general brain, no maturity.

Rick—specific brain (literature, philosophy, etc.), poise (on-stage, etc.), no "coolness" in person (awkward, in fact).

Linda—hidden brain (you'd almost never know), probably so-phisticated ideas but not sophisticated or a mover in practice.

I just looked at the Honor Roll list. I think I have the highest average of any girl in Advanced.

————————

I, too, felt that I was always just on the outskirts of the in-crowd, and I did not want to give up trying to infiltrate, either. I was staving off despair by staving off the recognition of my individuality. Perhaps I was taking my cues from my sister. Her individuality was giving her a lot of problems.

The year my parents said we would be moving, I had just entered junior high and felt like a big shot. I thought that if I could convince my parents I was truly miserable about having to leave what had been my only home, the move would not occur. I felt it unjust that such a major decision was being made without a unanimous vote.

On the morning of December 6, 1963, I sat in my bedroom holding on tightly to my cat as furniture was being removed from the house, piece by piece. Doren had left for school on the train that morning, overjoyed. She had been trying to con-vince me for weeks that I would love New York as much as she did. She would be there for me if I needed her because I would be attending the same school. But seventh grade at Walden was like sixth grade in my elementary school. You didn't move around from class to class—you stayed in one room. And at Walden I would be staying in one room with only twenty peo-ple—the entire seventh grade.

That first night in the apartment on Central Park West I couldn't have been more unhappy. Doren couldn't have been happier. My parents couldn't have been more harried. While the grown-ups busied themselves with unpacking, Doren and I sat in the empty bedroom that we would be sharing. Here I was, on the brink of adolescence, and Doren was in the thick of it. We had never shared a bedroom before, and this didn't seem to be a wonderful time to start. But we had no choice. The extra room, the "maid's room," my father had claimed as his study. Doren begged for that small space, but her plea was to no avail. My sister knew more of the impending disaster that would occur between us sharing a bedroom than I did.

Disaster did not strike right away. Doren was too happy

being a bona fide New Yorker to care at the outset about her sleeping quarters. Having Doren with me in the same room was no comfort. Our conflicting moods separated us. Doren was on a new voyage without me—she couldn't be held back and I wasn't ready to go along with her. New York had not been chosen for me, nor had the school I was attending. It was a school especially selected for Doren's needs, one that was specifically designed for "highly motivated" children. I was not one of those children. Academia was Doren's thing, not mine. Doren left trails of "A's" behind her; so as not to compete with such excellence, so as not to fail, I veered clear of those trails. In other words, I chose not to shine. At least not in the ways Doren had already staked out. The trouble was, she seemed to have claimed all possible avenues for shining. I was hard pressed to find my own way.

After her first day at Walden, Cathy came home crying, "It's dirty and ugly and I hate it." But I rejoice in the dirt. I am sick to death of immaculate suburbia. . . . The home of Walden is an ancient, dilapidated graystone—five floors plus a basement where the gym, art room, cafeteria, and staff lounge are located. The Lower School and Nursery are on the fifth floor (with access to the rooftop playground), the Middle School is on the fourth floor and some of the third, and the High School is on the third and second —mostly the second. Imagine—only one floor to accommodate an entire high school! . . . During the ten-minute breaks between classes, people sit on the long wooden bench in the second-floor lobby playing guitar, singing, reading, talking, flirting. A world apart from the hysterical 3 minute race between classes in my other school. . . . When the weather is good we use the breaks for a cigarette in Central Park. We sit on the railing at the entrance to the park—as many as six or seven can fit on the first section of it—and watch the Central Park West traffic go by. . . . When we have a free period—which happens a few times each week—we go to the drugstore on 86th Street for chocolate egg creams and French crullers. . . .

The girls in my class were wearing high heels. I bought myself a pair. They were wearing their long hair half up in a bun and half down. I bought bobby pins and did the same. They wore smock dresses and stockings. I adjusted my wardrobe. They all had pierced ears. The same jeweler that pierced their ears pierced mine. They all had boyfriends in the class. There were no boys left over for me. My entrance into the class made waves. I was the new kid on the block, I had red-blond hair down to my waist. I attracted attention. The boys flirted with me. The girls hated me.

Doren and I both needed attention from the opposite sex. We were not aware of how much energy we had spent as children trying to secure our father's attention and approval. Our unspoken theory was not an unusual one. If our father loved us, then how could he contemplate leaving us? We thought if we could secure our father's love, we would secure our parents' marriage. We mistook our father's disquiet with his life for disinterest in us. The fruitless challenge Doren and I devised did not die with our parents' separation. It became our task to transform the emotions of boys, and later men, from what appeared to be aloofness into attentiveness.

As the struggle to fit in began wearing me down, I set my sights on other territories—i.e., the boys in the higher grades. This made my sister nervous. The boys she brought home were looking at me a little too closely for her taste. And when she brought them home I hung around a little too long.

. . . I read some of my old journal to Cathy tonight and I think she is much younger at thirteen than I was—either that or she is much more secretive than I am. When I read her passages about Steve she asked, "How old were you when you first met him?" I was thirteen and he was eighteen. She said, "My God, that's like if I went out with Zev!" My stomach clutched. I can't begin to retell all the thoughts that passed through my mind simultaneously. Either Steve was incredibly young or I was incredibly old or Cathy is incredibly young or Zev is incredibly old. . . .

Of course the idea of Cathy having any real relationship with him is ridiculous, but somehow the whole idea threw me. . . .

Dream:

My sister had been hired by the Russian Ministry (somewhere in the country) to kill me because I was one of the dangerous people on their blacklist. They gave her three poisoned hypodermics and promised her $6,000 if she completed the job. Cathy tried to kill me twice but I was strong enough to fight her off. The third time I locked myself in the bathroom (parents') and screamed for my mother. She made Cathy give her the last needle. I couldn't decide whether I should confess to the Russians or just hide. I started to walk through Central Park to the ministry with my mother and Cathy trailing about 4 blocks behind me. The park was full of high school kids sprawled all over the grass. I became too scared to go because I thought they'd probably kill me themselves. I saw a boy I liked under a tree and fell upon him, my face buried in his stomach and my legs woven with his. . . . Just then a small, frail woman with reddish hair and brown skinny glasses came in front of us. I knew that she was a Russian agent searching out undesirables. I knew I'd be taken if I seemed to be a beatnik, so when she asked me questions I tried to act very proper. . . .

It wasn't long before the sign on our bedroom door went up: ENTER AT YOUR OWN RISK. Doren's handiwork. A divider was erected to separate the room in two. It was a mere pegboard, holes and all, hardly suitable for privacy. The Great Wall of China was what we needed.

Doren, as the older sister, chose the far side of the room, the side with the windows. My side was the one you had to walk through to get to the other side. My room doubled as a corridor for Doren and her visitors.

As our emotional division began to take hold, and rivalry began to take on a vivid life of its own, Doren and I found one thing we could share—the Beatles. One day as Doren was switching around on the AM dial, she suddenly yelped, "Cathy! You've got to listen to this song. Isn't it great? Shh-hhh! I've got to hear the words." I listened and I wasn't too crazy about this song that my sister was all red in the face about. Even so, I immediately thought that if Doren felt the song had merit, it must certainly have merit. The song was "I Wanna Hold Your Hand."

Shortly after this, Doren arrived home one day with the first Beatles album under her arm. She rushed into "our" bedroom and held it out in front of my face. "Okay," she said, "now tell me. Who do you think is the cutest of the four? I want your immediate response. No thinking. Just tell me quickly, which one do you think is the absolute cutest?" I was immediately anxious and sweating. This was a test. I pointed to a face on the album cover. It was George Harrison. Doren brought the album back against her chest and said simply, "No." I tried to hold my ground. "But that's who I think is the cutest. That one—" I grabbed the album away from her and pointed to George again. "No," Doren repeated, *"he's* the cutest"—she pointed at another face—"and his name is Paul. Paul is definitely the cutest. You picked George. He's not as cute as Paul. Paul is absolutely the *best Beatle.*" I didn't respond this time. I didn't argue. Doren was on her way to convincing me that Paul was to be my favorite Beatle. I don't know which was stronger—her powers of brainwashing or my acquiescence. But soon afterward I was writing my first love letter to Paul McCartney, buying my first Paul McCartney button, lying on the dining-room floor with my head between the stereo speakers listening to my favorite song sung by Paul McCartney. After all, Paul McCartney was the cutest and the best Beatle. Doren said so.

Sean and I arrived at Carnegie Hall quite early on the night of the concert and, since the early show was still on, we had to wait outside awhile. The crowd seemed about 75 percent female, the only guys being boyfriends like Sean who stood to lose their girls if they dared utter one disparaging word about the Beatles. . . .

Almost as soon as we got to our seats the show began, but it was only filler acts and some disc jockey in between revving up the audience—as if that were necessary—with questions like:

"Do you want the Beatles?"

A scream in unison: "Yes!"

"Awww, I don't think you really want the Beatles—that wasn't too loud. Now, c'mon. Do you want the Beatles? Let me hear it!"

Scream (hysterical now): "Yeeee-eeee-eeee-eeee-ssss!"

And after a few rounds with the disc jockey, the entire audience —me included—was prepared to loot, plunder, kill—anything— to prove the depth of our longing for the Beatles.

And then the magnificent four appeared. As they strode out to center stage to hook up their instruments, the air become combustible gas and their silvery, tight-suited bodies were the live matches that ignited the whole hall.

A scream went up—deafening and shrill—which rose in pitch as it increased in volume. And I was amused to discover that a scream was rising in my own throat; I had become one with the hysterical mob. This knowledge was both elating and terrifying.

Although the urge to scream was irresistible, it was temporarily checked by a disapproving look from Sean and a loudly whispered declaration that if I screamed he would lose all respect for me. To preserve Sean's precious respect (or the illusion that I needed to preserve it), I swallowed my latent jungle scream. . . .

I'm sure it's no exaggeration to state that for every fourteen, fifteen, or sixteen-year-old virgin present that night, this incredible group lust would long remain the paradigm of sexual experience.

I would not have been surprised if some member of the audience had run up on the stage in an attempt to copulate with one —or all—of the adored singers. One girl did try to jump out of her balcony seat and onto the stage, but an alert cop prevented her from carrying out the most significant act of her life.

At the end—when the Beatles were playing their encore—I realized that since all the cops were moving to the back of the theater in preparation for the exiting mob, there was nothing to stop me from going nearer the stage. I told Sean I was going to do it, and that there was nothing he could do to stop me. He said that if I went he would leave without me and, in addition, never speak to me again.

I walked briskly up to the stage and when I got there I smiled at Paul McCartney. And he smiled right back at me. Just like that. I was in ecstasy. There was surely enough joy for a lifetime concentrated in those three and a half minutes.

Needless to say, Sean didn't uphold his promise to abandon me. When I finally turned around to leave I bumped into him. I felt kind of sorry for him that night. . . . In the subway going home he asked me if I liked him as much as I liked Paul. I had to answer with the usual cop-out—that I liked them both in different ways. But I didn't like Sean one tenth as much. He could never make me that horny. Not in a million years.

I believed Doren to be graced with good fortune: she was always the one on the inside, I thought, whereas I remained on the outside looking in. Our experience regarding the first Beatles concert in New York—Doren was able to get tickets, I was not—further served to confirm my belief.

The alarm shocks me out of sleep at 5 A.M. The sleet is slamming down on the air conditioner and the wind is pouring in through the vents. The coldness of the bare wood floor travels up through my feet.

A pair of thick tights, two pairs of socks, weatherized boots, pants, and a couple of sweaters, and I'm ready. The heat is rising from the radiator as I fasten the hooks on the furry coat that makes me look like a stuffed gray bear.

The hallway is still dark and my parents' light is not shining through the crack under their bedroom door. I place my feet carefully, avoiding the spots that creak. I feel my way by touching the walls on either side of me, avoiding the low-hanging paintings. The thin stream of light flickering through the front-door peephole is my guide.

The sound of the elevator bell fills the hollow shaft, and I can hear the elevator man shuffling across the marble floor into the elevator.

"You're the first one up around here. You must have big plans."

Traveling down nine flights with him, I try to remember if we have given this one his Christmas tip.

"The Plaza Hotel, please. Oh, and could you go through the park?"

The cab driver skids around corners, slides through the powdered streets. The sleet is now snow and I examine individual snowflakes on the car window.

Close to 6 A.M. and already there are people sitting on the statue across from the Plaza. Some girls are huddled together in the statue's arms, others are up on her shoulders and head, or down in her lap, leaning against the statue's baby. Everyone is staring up at the left side of the hotel.

"Hey, what floor are they on?" someone yells, so I don't have to.

"Sixteen."

I join the three girls on the baby's head.

"Have you seen them yet?"

"No, but if you look up at—"

She is interrupted by a shriek. A girl on the shoulder above us is jumping up and down, her arms extended toward the sixteenth-story window.

"Paul! Paul! I saw him, I saw him! Oh my God, I saw him!"

There are intermittent cries of "Where?" "There! There!" She is pointing frantically toward a window. "Five from the left. Oh my God, it's him!"

I look up and don't know what I'm looking at but I think I see something, and maybe that something is Paul McCartney, so I scream with the rest of them, "Paul!"

6:30 A.M. and the crowd has thickened. I move with other girls to a side entrance of the hotel. We sit in closed-off streets, on police barriers and on curbs.

"I heard they came out of this door the other day," someone says.

By the afternoon I am making visits to the coffee shop around the corner to relieve my stinging limbs. After a while my body feels like it has been shot through with novocaine and I can't feel my face anymore. Since my body no longer seems to exist, the warmth of the coffee shop is no longer necessary.

Two hours before the concert the crowd begins to disperse. I missed out on getting tickets but I decide to go anyway. There is a crowd of people like me standing around Carnegie Hall. Someone whispers to me, "There's a way to get to their dressing room, wanna come with us?" Without a word, I follow a group that splits off from the rest.

I am on a fire escape. I hear my pants rip and feel slight pricks on my skin as I climb the rusty iron. Where the ladder ends, I use my hands to pull myself up to the next ledge.

We are inside Carnegie Hall on a dark floor and we press our ears against every door.

"Hey, you kids!"

The guards come after us.

Back on the fire escape, scrambling down the ladder, jumping on ledges, I hear myself screaming with the others.

7 P.M. My mother opens the front door and gasps. My pants are ripped at the ankles and knees, the stuffing is coming out of my jacket in various places, my hands are scratched and bloody, my hair is knotted and blown wild, my face is smeared with dirt. I don't know whether I'm laughing or crying. Neither does my mother.

Clean again, lying between newly washed sheets, I stare at the life-size poster of Paul on my wall before turning out the light. I don't want to be awake when my sister comes home, or if I am I don't want her to know I am. I don't want to hear how wonderful the concert was, how she got to see Paul, how I didn't.

Although we both became Beatle fanatics, Doren's enthusiasm was kept more in check than mine was. Doren did not, for example, cover her wall with Beatles posters. She did not climb up on top of a dresser every night to kiss Paul's face. Doren plastered her wall with photographs from *Vogue*, pictures of Jeanne Moreau, quotes by John Updike, *Playbill* covers, pictures of Marilyn Monroe, Barbra Streisand, Jonathan Miller, F. Scott Fitzgerald quotes, pictures of Oscar Werner, pictures of men and women embracing. Interspersed were some pictures of the Beatles, especially Paul. Her wall became so much a part of her identity that when she went off to college she took it with her—transferred it, picture by picture, quote by quote, onto mural-size paper. My Beatles wall eventually came down, was stored in cartons, and was replaced, mid-adolescence, by pictures of sunsets.

Staying out of each other's way was virtually impossible. We shared the same home, the same bedroom, the same school. . . . The question was, what *didn't* we share? There was something Doren had during that first year in New York that I didn't have—she was finally beginning to feel accepted by her peers. For the first time in her life she was starting to "fit in."

My status at Walden is superb. I am totally *in* with THE GROUP. I mean now they ask *me* what *I* want to do and will *I* come with *them*. I have to admit I don't find it unpleasant. Scholastically—my teachers are all raving about me. I really shine in French (and History and English and Math) and I'm on the top in Chemistry. . . . Stan T., who I'll have for Math next year, knows all about me, and when I asked him what he thought about early admissions he said, "Don't do it. I want to teach you." My ego, needless to say, has never been in better shape. . . . I haven't been writing. I simply have nothing to say. Nothing is driving me insane, in other words. My father has been keeping away, school is fine and occasionally a lot of fun. I hardly see my mother or sister, etc. What's more, I like myself (in general). I AM ALL RIGHT. . . .

I became friends with Cleo one day in early spring, passing notes during History class re her encounter with Andy Warhol. Warhol wanted Cleo to be in one of his movies (she has that little girl-little boy look), but she turned him down because she got the impression (undoubtedly correct) that his "factory" is into hard drugs.

Since the first day of our friendship, Cleo and I have talked of nothing but finding lovers—preferably one for each of us, but not necessarily different ones since we're such good friends, and since we didn't dare hope to fall in love "in time." In time for what?

Why, in time to prevent us from reaching June and graduation with virginity intact.

Well, Cleo doesn't have to worry anymore.

She phoned yesterday afternoon in an ecstasy of whispers and giggles and answered the inevitable question of the uninitiated ("How WAS it?") with a confused silence and then, "Well, uh, I don't know. Strange. Wow. I kept thinking it was going to push through my body and come out of my mouth. Weird."

I was duly impressed. . . .

―――――――――

As for me, contentment was not any part of my experience. My ego was on the lookout for a boost. Of course it had to be a male boost. There was a boy in the class who I had no interest in. His girlfriend was the class ringleader, a young lady to be reckoned with. But one day I heard, via the whispered grapevine, that he liked me. Poof! Like magic, I set my sights on him. My intentions were kept secret and ultimately were to no avail save one dance at a class party. Perhaps it had been a faulty grapevine. As far as I could tell, there was no member of the opposite sex at Walden who liked me. I found out almost twenty years later that I was wrong about that—from someone who had been Doren's classmate, one of the boys she used to invite home. "We were all infatuated with you," he informed me. Gene and I had re-met and spent time together during the last weeks Doren was alive. "You were the beautiful, mysterious blonde. We all made bets on who was going to get to you first." I was shocked by this information at thirty and would have been even more startled had I known at the time. Doren was the beautiful, mysterious creature. I was only in her shadow. How could anyone have noticed me at all?

―――――――――

My sister is a little pain in the ass now that she thinks she is a woman in her own right and all that. She pesters me when boys are around, when they're not she moans how barren and desperate her life has become and right now she has two horrible gossipy girlfriends here who are definitely not lessening my tremendous sense of anxiety. . . .

―――――――――

To top off my sense of being a stranger in the company of any person or in any environment, I was suddenly perversely blessed with my first period. The event elicited my mother's tenderness, my father's nervousness, and my sister's wrath. I didn't understand why. It was bad enough that now my body was a stranger to me as well. The bleeding came on with such a vengeance that I was in bed for the first day with severe cramps. Doren scolded me. "Get out of bed!" she yelled. "What's the matter with you?! It's *only* your period, for God's sake! Why are you making it such a big deal? Christ! I can't believe you're lying there in bed!" I heard loud voices all around me that day. Doren yelled at me, and my mother yelled at Doren, trying to protect me from her verbal assaults. I felt ill, and apparently Doren felt exceedingly uneasy herself. It might "only" have been my period, it might only have been the most natural thing in the world . . . but another transition was taking place, one which meant Doren was perhaps on the way to losing her little baby sister. And perhaps, too, on her way to gaining a bona fide competitor. How was she going to fulfill her role as my protector now? How was she going to keep me safe?

Doren spent as much time away from home as possible. She resented anything or anyone that might impede her independence. More and more I saw her in the company of Zev, the much revered senior at Walden. Every girl in school had a crush on him. Including me. I felt privileged in that he spent some time at our house and I was able to report back to my female classmates new details about this person we were all having severe fantasies about. He looked like Paul McCartney.

I start by remembering Zev, and discover without too much surprise that the image of him crossing the street to go into the park, or perched on the wrought-iron fence dispassionately observing Gene's W. C. Fields routine (complete with white gloves) for maybe the two hundredth time, is still fresh. . . . And I begin the long-familiar analysis to explain why—first, of course, is the way he looked, ordinary in the extreme: black jeans, generally, slightly too short due to the shrinkage incurred in relentless launderings by his mother; a drab army-surplus jacket, worn indoors and outdoors regardless of season; under that a nearly colorless sweater, often a thin beige one; and, after girls started to stop him on the street to inquire if he was John Lennon or Paul McCartney, often a heavy black turtleneck, which made the resemblance slightly stronger—at least to the John or Paul of the first official photograph of the Beatles published in America in *Mademoiselle* (pronounced maa-dimisel by its readers) magazine. . . .

And his ambiguous, inanimate face, which once or twice a week might smile at me in an astonishing gesture of goodwill. . . .

Straining for her autonomy, Doren grew more and more defiant. Instead of helping to appease turmoil in the family, she began to be its overt cause. Doren decided it was just not conceivable that she observe the curfew that had been set for her. She began staying out very late, way past her assigned deadline. And then it wasn't long before she would leave home in the evening and not return until the following day. No matter that every time she did this, my mother would be catapulted into dread fear that something drastic, and most likely fatal, had occurred, and my father would erupt into a white-hot rage over Doren's disobedience. I would plead with my sister to control her aberrant behavior. Didn't she care about the tremendous upheaval she was stirring up? She refused to talk about it. It wasn't until we were adults that Doren acknowledged she felt out of control. "Cathy," she said, "I just couldn't help myself. I *knew* I was causing trouble and that the tension in the house was escalating because of it. I not only couldn't help myself, I didn't even feel guilty. Not coming home at night gave me a thrill—even knowing what I would have to face the next morning."

David had a party last night to celebrate the departure of his parents to Europe for a one-month trip. It was a glorious party—gloriously high—from the initial three rounds of Brandy Alexanders through the passing of the pot at 3:00 A.M., and right into dawn.

I decided to stay through the morning, hazarding the wrath of my parents in the hope that an 8:30 A.M. call home to let them know I was all right would minimize my punishment. But my father called at 7:00 A.M.—in a rage—and commanded my immediate return. I coolly told him I would be home at 9:00 sharp and hung up.

To avoid an early morning fight, I went to sleep the minute I got back, but there was a showdown in the kitchen at 2:30 this afternoon when my father demanded a list of the names of the people at the party so he could "make trouble for them." Naively, I asked him what he was trying to prove, and with one fell swoop he sent brunch—bagels and lox, dishes and cups of coffee, and the electric coffeepot too—flying to the floor. Some of the boiling coffee landed on my mother and me.

My mother started to shriek, in pain and anger, an effect which brought my sister to some sort of critical mass, and she called my father a bastard to his face. Then my father hit my sister, producing a quite awesome nosebleed, and my mother hit him, and I stood convulsed with fear in a far corner of the kitchen.

Now my father is locked into his study; my mother is still in the kitchen, sobbing and pleading for her dead father's assistance, clutching my sister, who is wailing uncontrollably; and I'm hiding in my bedroom with no intention of exiting in the near future.

Another Sunday. There is the smell of bacon and I hear voices in the kitchen. I pull the quilt over my head and try to ignore that I am awake, that I'll soon be hungry, that it will be impossible to sleep through Sunday.

I sit quietly outside the kitchen, listening for information —what time my sister came home last night, if my father saw her coming in late, and if I have missed another scene. I want to know exactly what the situation is before becoming a part of it. I want to determine Sunday before it happens.

All appears to be quiet. I peek around the corner. My sister is sitting by the window, staring into her cereal bowl, filling the spoon with milk, then letting it spill out again. Her hair falls on either side of her face. My mother is at the stove staring at the kettle filled with water, waiting for it to whistle. I walk into the kitchen and sit down across from my sister. I wait for her to look up at me. She doesn't.

"Doren came home late again. Your father wouldn't listen to me. He's going to punish her." My mother's voice is calm, defeated. Doren looks up now. Her face is red and blotchy from crying. I hear the closet door in my parents' bedroom slam shut. I wish I had never left my bed and warm quilt.

"Cathy," Doren says, "please don't go. Stay with me." She looks down again into her bowl.

"Doren, why don't you just come home when you're supposed to? Aren't you sick of this already?" I'm angry. "Why do you keep doing this?"

The floor creaks from the weight of my father's steps through the hall. It seems like he makes it to the kitchen in four giant strides. The cat's ears and tail stiffen, and she runs, sideways, out of the room. I laugh nervously. The vein above my father's left eye is visible. He pulls the plastic container of orange juice out of the refrigerator and slams it on the table. I cover my ears with my hands.

"You'll never learn, will you, Doren!" His voice cracks. Doren gasps, my mother stands motionless at the sink. "Answer me!" He raises his voice another octave, and his face is almost purple. Doren screams, "Stop it!" but does not look up. My father hurls the orange juice across the table. I jump up and clutch my mother. With my head buried in her waist, I scream, "Shut up! Shut up! Shut up!" over and over again. The table is overturned. "Bastard!" I yell. Now I hear only bits of what my father is screaming: "ignorant . . . ungrateful . . . guttersnipe. . . ." I hurl myself at him, pummeling him on his arms with my fists. Doren and my mother pull me away. I feel something hard across my face that forces me back. Doren is sitting on the floor, pointing at my face. I put my hand to my nose and then look at blood on my fingers. My father disappears. Doren holds my hand. "Don't be afraid," she says, crying, "I'm sorry."

It is now quiet. I listen hard to an unfamiliar muffled sound. It is coming from behind a closed door. It is my father sobbing.

My mother knew my father better than I did. She knew that what had happened was an accident, that he had not meant to hurt me. She wanted me to go to him, to forgive him. The blame, she felt, should not be put on him but rather on a strained marriage that both of them were trying to find the courage to get out of. But even though I trusted her, I chose not to relinquish my anger. It was too difficult to maintain a consistent anger at Doren. I still needed her too much. It didn't occur to me to be angry at my mother. In fact I did not experience adolescent rebellion until I was well into my twenties. The person I could most easily blame for my discomfort in the world was my father. I felt like a victim, so I had to point my finger at someone.

I blamed Lori Barton for being a kleptomaniac and stealing my favorite blue change purse when we were five years old. I blamed her for not confessing. I blamed the hairdresser who cut all my hair off when I was six and who told me how adorable I was going to look with a pixie haircut. I blamed my mother for making me come out of my room after three days instead of letting me stay inside until my hair grew long enough to cover my ears. I blamed my sister for totally disappearing during a game of hide-and-seek and then telling me the wind took her away to a castle in the sky. I blamed her for not asking the wind to take me too. I blamed the wind for sometimes carrying with it the smell of The Fog Man. When we lived in Merrick I was terrified of the man in the little red truck that came around during the summer to kill insects. A dense white cloud of toxic smoke would pour out of the back of the truck. When I would smell The Fog Man and I would be too far from home to make it there in time before being enveloped by the poisonous white cloud, I'd pound on people's doors, begging for them to let me in, to protect me from The Fog Man. I blamed them for their mock smiles, for sending me home, for telling me there was nothing to be afraid of, The Fog Man wouldn't harm me, for suggesting that I play in the smoke like the other children. I would have to run like a demon, faster than the demon pursuing me, take all the shortcuts, hold my breath until I made it into the house, slam and lock the door behind me, stand on the coffee table to close all the blinds in the living room. I'd curl myself into the couch and lie in the dark room, waiting.

My fear and insecurity were so amorphous, I had to find targets of explanation. After I no longer had The Fog Man, my father became the substitute. We became one another's enemy. Doren, on the other hand, needed our father in a way from which I had extricated myself. At least I thought I had. I pretended for a long time that I didn't have a father. Doren didn't do this. She would often tell me how relaxed and loving our father was during her early years, before I was born. Doren had experienced a special kind of warmth and openness with our father, and she would always continue to seek out with him what she had experienced as a young child. She would not give up on him. I, on the other hand, did—for a long while. And we both paid for our decisions.

I avoided Doren at school because she would always introduce me to her friends as her "little sister," or sometimes even "baby sister." I would subsequently get teased by the boys in Doren's class. They'd follow me down the hallway, chanting, "There goes Doren Arden's baby sister." What I didn't know is that they were flirting with me. If I had been aware of it at the time, I would have been flattered instead of tortured. As it seemed then, my status as Doren Arden's sister was not doing me any good whatsoever so it wasn't exactly something I cared to advertise.

As I worked to get a good hate going toward my sister, as

the reverse was also true, she had the audacity to come down with a case of blood poisoning. This was actually not so different as something I felt, twenty years later, when she got cancer. I would be angry at her then as well, she had been intruding in my life in ways I did not appreciate and I let her know that I wanted nothing to do with her, that what I in fact wanted was a bona fide estrangement. And then she got cancer.

But, that first year in New York City, it was blood poisoning that drew me back to the loving fold. There was a blister on the back of her heel, caused by a tight shoe. A young, rambuctious child had stomped on her foot, smashing the blister and causing an infection. Doren had not realized it. She had gone to the doctor for another minor ailment when he discovered a blue line traveling up her leg. It was already almost up to her knee. I don't know if Doren was aware of the seriousness of her condition, but it was clear the doctor impressed the danger upon my mother. He developed some concoction and a way of bathing Doren's foot every hour over a period of twenty-four hours.

Doren was in pain. It was my first introduction to watching my sister in physical agony. She lay in bed with the bad foot, swathed in cloths and plastic Baggies, out of the covers. The procedure the doctor had written out for my mother to perform on the wound necessitated staying up all night. I don't know if my mother actually slept at all that night, or if she was setting an alarm to go off every hour. But she was in our room every hour on the minute.

Although I could have stayed in my bed while my mother administered to Doren, I became a partner in the healing process. The solution would already be prepared when Mother came in. She would begin to bathe Doren's foot and I would then help her wrap it up again in warm cloths and plastic. Every hour I examined the blue line on Doren's leg to see if it was traveling up or downhill. During this hourly ritual, all of us were relatively silent. There was a job to be done. Doren lay back with her eyes closed, wincing back pain as she would many years later, allowing my mother and me to take care of her. During that night the bond among all of us had to do with trust. My mother was fully confident we would help Doren to heal. This confidence guided us all. Doren's faith in her own healing powers came second. My faith came last. I could trust my mother's confidence and her motherly healing powers, but I was not yet at the point where I could have that kind of faith in myself and my own abilities. What I remember more than anything else was my nervous stomach. The next day I reluctantly went to school and thought only about Doren. I was scolded in gym class for inattention. Doren was the center of my world that day, as she would be during the two and a half years of her fatal illness. I wasn't aware during those twenty-four hours just how concerned I really was, or how frightened, or how bonded I was to my sister. That kind of daze would later come back to me. And, later, it would envelop my entire world for years.

The blue line did recede. Doren did recover. In some way I was relieved to know I had had a hand in that recovery. It was a change from feeling powerless. I had connected with my sister in a way that was not altogether dependent. It opened up another avenue that would allow the dependency to change hands. A new part was added to the old system. It would take a long time to trust its efficiency, so by no means were we foolhardy enough to throw out the familiar, rusty machine.

It is late at night. I am ready to go to sleep. When I turn my light off Doren's light shines through the little holes of the brown divider that separates us. I position myself in bed so I can peek through one of the peg-board holes. Doren is in her bed surrounded by books and papers. She is cutting up one piece of paper and Scotch-taping it to another. She is very careful to cut evenly. Every once in a while she takes a sip of iced tea but does not seem to stop concentrating as she sips. Doren has been in this same position all day, writing a paper. Only once did she get up in the after-noon to make herself a grilled-cheese sandwich with tomato. I am too tired to watch her for very long and as my eyes close I think about how it is a given that Doren will get an "A" on any paper she writes. This one is on Hermann Hesse. I would be very grateful if she'd finish her work and turn out her light because it is shining in my eyes through those damn holes.

It is a silent weekday meal, the four of us around the table for dinner. The housekeeper, who comes in once a week, has made my favorite fried chicken. I am grateful for the silence because the opposite of that is someone being reprimanded for something. Last night it was Doren for being lax about drying dishes. We all have our places to go after eating. Doren will go into the bedroom to do her homework, which she always does in bed. Mother will retire to her bedroom, will fall asleep by 8 P.M., and before nine the phone will ring and she will talk to a friend for hours. My father will retire to his study and I won't see him until to-morrow night at dinner. I will go into the dining room, watch television until eleven, get ready for bed, then go into my closet, turn on the overhead closet light, close the closet door, pull out my journal (hidden among winter sweaters on a top shelf), sit down on the extra kitchen chair I have confiscated—and I will write.

*W*e thought perhaps we'd be something akin to the Brontë sisters—world-famous sisters who write and who would be remembered and read way past their lifetimes. Actually it was Doren who first had this fantasy and spoke about it. We were both in our twenties. It would amuse me to hear, and I'd chime in with her scenario, but I never actually believed it. That is because Doren was The Writer. Not I. Ever since my second-grade play, when I performed the role of Slinky the Witch and won the accolades of an entire school with my evil ways, I was The Actress. I don't know when it was that Doren received her designation, but she was always my sister who was The Writer.

When I began to write consistently at thirteen, I had no inclination to want to share that writing with anyone. How could I dare set words on paper when my sister was so brilliant at the same thing? No one must know, I thought. And not because I felt my writing would have no place within the family belief system, but because I was running scared from the competition. Doren was good, and I could never hope to be as good. I was compelled to write, but I was also compelled to keep it to myself.

So it was just me and my closet. I loved that closet in much the same way I now love my first car. Both liberated me. My closet had a green linoleum tile floor, lots of room for clothes and shoes and me and a chair. The pièce de résistance was the light with a pull chain on the ceiling. What luxury! Not for my wardrobe, but for me and my journal.

For a while no one knew about my sanctuary. I'd disappear in there during family arguments, or in the middle of the night when everyone was asleep, or just when I needed privacy and also needed to write. Eventually my family caught on. When I couldn't be found they knew where I was. I would often hear someone say "Where's Cathy?" and someone respond "Oh, she's in her closet." If I ever said I was writing in there, I mumbled it under my breath. If my writing in the closet was ever acknowledged, it was in the most offhand, casual, disinterested way. "Oh, I don't know, she's in there writing or something." That was the attention my writing received in our house. It was always an "or something."

It was Doren who guessed I was keeping a journal. Since she had been keeping one for years, this was nothing unusual to her. She was pleased, in fact, that I was doing something other than being interested in boys and going to parties and watching *The Tonight Show* and *Hullabaloo*. She made me swear I would never read her journal. It made me uncomfortable that I knew where it was, right there in the top drawer of her purple dresser. I didn't understand why she just didn't hide it like me and not take the chance of some nosy person losing control. Of course, I was that nosy person. There were a few times when no one was home that I just couldn't bear to stay away from that drawer. It might as well have had flashing lights on it for how conspicuous it was to me. If I actually read anything, it was for two minutes, and then I was so coiled with fear and guilt that I would never remember anything I had seen. How could I not be compelled to take a glance now and again at the writing that was keeping me holed up in my closet?

All of Doren's journals were eventually before me. Twenty-four hours after she died I was helping to pack up everything in her apartment. I remember the bookshelves most of all—I pulled out one loose-leaf notebook after the other. I held on to them before transferring them to cartons, staring at the red cover, the blue cover, the black cover, amazed at how much writing was there and that Doren's deepest feelings and private thoughts were now in my hands.

Even though Doren and I were scrambling for our respective independence, Doren's mothering feeling didn't end. She frequently talked about wanting her own baby. If only the day would come when she could be a mother, she thought, so many of her problems would be solved. Doren's craving to want to nurture was one that grew in its compelling nature throughout her life. The summer after we had moved to Manhattan, she discovered a fulfilling outlet for these emotions. She was overjoyed. Doren would rediscover this form of giving during the last year of her life. It would become more gratifying for her than writing.

What a difference a day makes. My plans for summer 1963 are almost settled. I'm not going back to Trebor. I'm going to work at Brookville with mentally retarded children. I feel relieved and terribly excited. . . .

The night Cathy left for camp I dreamt she died. . . . Her ghost was visible only to me so I took her with me everywhere and people became curious as to why I would talk to air. I remember feeling guilty because the burden of her ghost was unpleasant to me. . . .

I had an unusual dream last night. I dreamt I had a baby. The whole thing is pretty vague, but this I remember: I was calm about the whole thing and almost happy. . . . I told my father. He got angry . . . and I remember being *stunned*. I actually did not understand how anyone could be angry because I had a baby. . . . And before I woke up I had a satisfied feeling. As if I'd accomplished something very worthwhile. . . .

Tomorrow is *it*. I have butterflies. Oh please, God, let me be good. Let it be right. . . .

. . . I'm very proud of myself, and I feel important. I can handle some of the kids better than the old-timers. . . . I *adore* work. It's a remarkable and exhausting experience.

Donna got on my nerves today a little. On Monday her left leg was a little bad, on Tuesday her left leg and left arm were bad, today she acted like she was paralyzed. It was murder to get her out of the pool.

I've been feeling very maternal lately. I suppose I'm "getting ready for motherhood"?

. . . Ingrid came out in a bikini and Joe, a counselor I'm attracted to, was fooling around with her. He came back to me, however. THANK GOD. I'm so terrified he'll lose interest. . . . I feel mother(ly) and lover(ly). . . .

When I was with Cathy today (visitors day at Trebor) I got the strangest feeling. Somehow my emotions and thoughts about Joe got mixed up with her and for a minute I couldn't figure out our relationship. *For a minute I thought she was Joe!* It was awful. . . .

This summer I learned how deeply rewarding it is to give and, for the first time in my life, I felt useful. . . .

In eighth grade I started feeling like a big shot. Finally I no longer was confined to one classroom with one teacher. Now I was privileged and had many teachers and many classrooms. The biggest bonus of all was that my grade was no longer isolated on the third floor, away from all the big-kid action. We were now on the second floor. This was the moment I had been waiting for. High school.

When I entered high school Doren was in the graduating class. So, as usual, she was a bigger shot than me. It seemed that the boys in her class were the cutest in the entire school.

And the especially cutest were the ones who found their way to our house. They were Doren's territory, however, so I decided the next to the cutest boys were located in the tenth grade.

Doren was glad to have me out of the way once I began to be socially active. But somehow I still seemed to be around when Doren would arrive home with a cutie. I was definitely attracted to the boys she was attracted to, though it never occurred to me that there was any competition. I just knew she didn't want me around.

One of the attributes Doren and I always prided ourselves on was that we could never be interested in the same man. We thought this was very lucky, that our tastes ran differently. How this misconception came to be, I don't know.

> . . . you'll never guess who I saw on Columbus Avenue! Zev! He smiled and said Hi. I thought I would die! He never *ever, ever* says Hi to anyone! When I told Doren he said Hi to me, she was very shocked. . . . He looked *great* today!

> After I got home, Doren came home with Zev. He's been very nice to me. I think Doren thinks he likes me.

> When I got out of school I saw Zev across the street in the park. Doren came out of school so I started walking across the street with her. . . . Zev asked Doren if she wanted to go for a soda at Lido's. Then he asked me if I wanted to come so I said, "Yes, but I won't because I don't think Doren wants me." I then walked away with my friends. When I returned home Zev and Doren were going into the dining room. Zev asked, "Do you want to come in with us?" I smiled, and he smiled.

> Zev called at about 8:15 tonight, but Doren was at the Philharmonic. . . . I love him.

> Whenever I look at myself in the mirror I get very upset. I just don't look like the likable type. First of all I'm too tall, and since my hair is long and flat on my head, my head looks too small for my body. I wish I knew if anyone liked me. I'm so confused, it's disgraceful!

My writing remained a secret, as did my interest in boys. Not just Doren's boys, but also my own. Doren's interest in both areas, on the other hand, was apparent. Her papers and stories that always came back with "A's" were read and discussed with our parents, and praised. Her interest in boys, while not praised, was at least recognizable: Doren brought her boyfriends home. I didn't bring a boyfriend home until I was thirty. Doren was intent on getting approval about whoever it was she brought home. If I had received a family member's approval about a boy I was going out with, I would have stopped going out with him.

Even given the undercurrent of competition, the approval Doren most coveted was from her little sister. She may have been uneasy that I hung around Zev and her too often, but she was pleased to know I approved of him. From the early days one of the family myths that had been perpetuated was that Cathy was a "witch." If Doren was considered the one with the brains, I was considered the one with the intuition. I assumed that according to my family, intuition had nothing to do with brains.

Zev ran hot and cold with Doren. She finally gave up her quest for consistent attention and committed love from him. But the quest, in its own right, continued. After Zev was gone, Doren met someone who renewed her faith in requited love. She had met Peter through his two closest friends, Allyn and Jamie. The three young men were a tight threesome. After assessing the situation for a while, Doren finally settled on Peter.

I met a guy at a party who talked a great deal about his idyllic childhood. I was pretty uninterested until he said that his favorite records as a child were "Celeste" and "Tubby the Tuba." That startled me because they were my favorites too.

His name is Allyn.

Met Allyn's incredibly attractive friend Jamie, who's already been accepted by Hamilton. I can't have anything except one good minute—if that—with him.

Allyn's so jealous he tries to keep me away from parties and, if we do happen to go to one, he becomes incensed if I wear anything but jeans and T-shirt.

A few weeks ago he was racked with fear because Jamie had told him that he was "enchanted" with me. And now Allyn's friend Peter owes me a dollar . . . and since Peter wants to return it personally, Allyn is afraid that Peter, too, desires me. . . .

Allyn phoned tonight to tell me that Peter was very depressed about finally breaking up with Susan and would I mind very much if he came with us to see *The Pawnbroker*. I had to conceal my glee.

As usual, Allyn made a fool of himself. While we were waiting in the lobby before the show, he bent down to pick up a candy bar he had dropped and those contraceptives he's always reminding me about fell out of his jacket pocket and onto the floor for all the multitudes to see.

Naturally, several people in the lobby noticed and recognized the package on the floor before Allyn scrambled awkwardly to return it to the inside pocket of his jacket. There followed several minutes of ridicule in the form of titters and hilarious glances. . . .

Before the movie began I sandwiched myself between Allyn (on my left) and Peter (on my right). By the end of the movie the vibrations to and from my right were ecstatically strong.

I like the threeness. I'm really in trouble.

Jamie has suddenly, and inexplicably, decided to hate me.

During a lull at a recent party he turned to me and said contemptuously, "I hear you're hated at Walden."

It took me a second to regain my balance, but then I countered with, "And I hear you're loathed at E.I." (his school)

Everyone laughed their approval of my parry, but I felt disgraced for the rest of the evening.

Last Sunday night Peter called me on a pretext (to speak to Allyn) and we talked for three hours. Before the conversation was over we had cautiously sounded each other out, discovered and proclaimed our mutual affection.

Tonight I broke up with Allyn. He gave me the "Jules et Jim" record I've been searching for for more than a year and some angry, Magic Marker letters to maintain his dignity. . . .

Also: there was a tiny paper and toothpick "Peace" flag stuck right through the record jacket. When I unwrapped the gift I was dismayed to find a hole in Jeanne Moreau's left cheek.

I love Peter. This is not a whim.

Before Doren brought Peter home, any other young man she had brought into the house I had sized up within minutes and shared with her my brief synopsis. If I said "Yea," she'd have hope the relationship would proceed well. If I said "Nay," or forecasted danger, Doren would then expect it. In the case of Peter, I wholeheartedly approved. I also wholeheartedly developed a crush on him. Doren was aware of it, but now it didn't seem to bother her. She thought it was cute. She did fear Peter's betrayal, as we both feared betrayal from anyone of the opposite sex, but this time that fear was not projected onto me.

————————

Late at night before Peter rushes to the Port Authority to get the last bus back to North Bergen, we have a pretty good amount of privacy. I've even learned my apartment by touch so that after Peter leaves I can noiselessly make my way back to my bedroom in the dark.

But the quality of our intimacy on Friday and Saturday nights is fast deteriorating, mostly owing to the lurid three-sectioned couch, which is the only piece of furniture nearly bedlike in the entire den. I'm certain that my father planned it that way—he isn't about to lose sleep worrying about his daughter's virtue so he lets the couch do his work for him. Peter was good humored at first, but his patience is waning. We can't even kiss each other without the couch sliding in three directions. . . .

Peter will work in a paint factory for the next four weeks, then vacation in Europe for eight weeks, and next fall he will leave for Berkeley. . . . I try to accept the imminence of summer, fall, and winter separations. . . .

————————

When Doren was in the den with the door closed and Peter in there with her, I guessed what was going on. But I couldn't believe she had the courage to fool around when there were other people in the house. I would never think about bringing anyone home unless the place was vacant.

The apartment promised to be a bit more vacant when Doren left for college. She had applied to five of the Seven Sister schools. Her first choice was Radcliffe, and this put her in competition with Ellen, another girl in her class. Radcliffe would not accept both of them. Doren had been in competition with her ever since arriving at Walden. Not just academically, but socially as well.

For some reason, I link together Doren's learning how to drive and her waiting for word from Radcliffe. They were happening at the same time and she was extremely uncomfortable at both. My father had recently bought a gold sports car, and although Doren liked the idea of being behind the wheel, she was miserable doing it. My father was taking her out for lessons. When they returned from one of these lessons they wouldn't speak to each other or anyone else for two days at least. I went out with Doren myself, for the fun of it, when she had acquired a learner's permit. Once again, the idea of driving off in a car with my sister was a heavenly notion, but the reality didn't match the fantasy. I went driving around the neighborhood with her once, she hit a car while trying to park, cursed at every intersection, and yelled at me when I attempted assistance. The excursion was a lot of things, but it was by no means heavenly and it was my first and last rendezvous with Doren as chauffeur. Doren managed to get her license, but she never drove again. Never.

So coupled with the tension of learning how to drive was the tension of acceptance or rejection from Radcliffe. She was appeased when she received an acceptance letter from Bryn Mawr. Her relief was only temporary.

I've been accepted early by Bryn Mawr and I'm the envy of all my classmates, including Ellen. . . . Of course we both wait with bated breath for April, when it will be known which of us Radcliffe prefers. . . .

When Doren received a rejection from Radcliffe she was devastated. She had always excelled, been the best, never had had to compete academically before this. It must have felt to her that she was losing her grip on the one aspect of her life she had always been able to rely on. Hardly a mention of her defeat went into the journal, except as a parenthetical statement—"(Ellen got into Radcliffe)." She cried for a long time and then called Ellen to congratulate her.

I didn't think very much about Doren's impending departure. What I did do was form an attachment to a counselor at my camp in Maine. Doren had stopped going to Trebor the summer before. This counselor, Susan, became as important to me as Doren. The following summer I found out just before going to camp that Susan would not be returning. I felt utter loss and helplessness. It was easier directing these feelings toward Susan rather than my sister. When I arrived at camp I quickly became attached to the music counselor, Lesley. I don't remember missing Doren at all. At the end of that summer I wrote in my journal, about Lesley—"I don't want her to forget me. Ever. I'll never forget her."

I returned home to Doren's departure.

Well, Doren is gone. It doesn't really seem like she isn't here. I don't know why. The divider is down and the room is rearranged. Maybe it hasn't hit me yet.

I love that phrase, "The divider is down." As if by magic, divine intervention, anything but my own hand. The fact is I almost killed myself dismantling that divider, and I must have accomplished the task in record time. The process of making the bedroom mine alone commenced immediately.

The room was huge. I could see the windows. I could walk to the far end and not get scolded. I could close the bedroom door and be ALONE. Hello, privacy; goodbye, closet. If my father had not forbidden it, I would have put a lock on the bedroom door. The idea that anyone could walk in on me while I was writing still filled me with dread. I continued to write in my journal late at night when my parents were asleep. After Doren left I cried often but couldn't identify the source of my unhappiness.

_____

Elizabeth and I spotted each other instantly in our first few hours at Bryn Mawr and conversed in somewhat hysterical tones till the wee hours of our first night there. We hid out on the wide terrace behind Rhoads Hall while the rest of the dorm underwent the ordeal of the first Hall Meeting. The knowledge that I was beginning my college career by breaking a rule (attendance at the meeting had been declared compulsory) had filled me with a warm sense of security. I suspected Elizabeth was invulnerable to the vicissitudes of life at school and felt confident some of her invulnerability would rub off on me. . . .

Elizabeth doesn't care for Candice and the feeling is mutual. This makes things extraordinarily difficult for me. . . . I like both of them. . . .

Candice and I have become so fed up with the lack of privacy in the bathroom we have resorted to standing guard for each other whenever possible. It's not difficult for either of us to keep girls away—most of the girls on our corridor are terrified of us anyway, since we've made it clear we disdain small talk of any kind, be it about the terrible quality of the food or the degree of excellence or lack of excellence of one professor or another.

The first mixer of the year was scheduled to be held in the gymnasium on our first Friday at school. It goes without saying that every dormitory was in a collective frenzy from sunrise to sunset—girls showering, bathing, drying and setting hair, chattering, drinking gallons of Cokes and consuming pounds of potato chips, blasting records and dancing solo to get in the party spirit.

Candice was in a foul mood all day because she had suddenly realized that all her skirts and dresses were a full four inches longer than anyone else's and she had set about to shorten immediately every offending item in her wardrobe in order to prevent her peers from branding her old-fashioned.

Elizabeth was calm, but expectant. Eddie and she had decided that she ought to stay at school at least for her first weekend—to see if there were any people around who might be qualified to be her friends—especially any guys who might like to be her escort on weekends when she couldn't be in New York with Eddie, but who would not make any sexual demands on her. (Eunuchs?)

Elizabeth is faring much better than I am, but not really because she's stronger, although she may be. She has her personal life under control (screwing weekends only) and so there is nothing to prevent her from working hard and well during the week.

Right now she is into the pre-Socratic philosophers so she doesn't talk about much besides Pythagoras, Heraclitus, Empedocles, and, of course, Eddie. . . . She relates to me in detail the course of her affair. . . . But she seems to take inordinate pleasure in telling me about Eddie's social triumphs (most notably his new friendship with Jasper Johns)—a fact that causes me to believe her emotional interest in him is on the wane. . . .

Elizabeth is no more moody than when we first became friends, but she often drops hints about her more secret hurts. Last night she showed me a little article on page 16 of *The New York Times* about the separation of her parents—her mother and stepfather. Her mother has a fairly prominent government job. She bitterly told me that if she hadn't picked up the paper, she never would have known about it. Although I could sympathize with her position, it seemed rather glamorous to me to be able to read family news in the *Times*.

Elizabeth has long claimed to have written me notes that I have never seen. Last week the reason became clear: She writes them on facial tissue.

I realized this one night as I was about to blow my nose into a tissue that read "GO TO BED SILLY."

Now that I'm wise to her medium, I'm sorry to say her notes are generally cover-ups for borrowing something or other.

For example: "Dearest Doren, Your room is lovely this way. . . . Thanks very much for the suitcase. I promise to take good care of it. . . ." Or: "Doren-luv, Took your phil notebook (I couldn't or didn't get up for class)—also took *Rubber Soul*. Can you come to my room for both of them after dinner?"

———————

This first year that Doren was away I developed a powerful infatuation with a very handsome, very withholding young man, Mark. I was not the only young lady interested in Mark. He had quite a following. I was heartsick and smack dab in the middle of fierce competition. I hated the situation, but was obviously compelled by it as well. The journey Doren and I were both on—trying to derive attention from an inattentive male—was a frustrating one, but titillating nonetheless.

I would write to Doren about my Mark dilemma, and she would write to me about her Peter dilemma. She felt college would be all right if only Peter were with her and not in Berkeley. In all Doren's letters she referred to me as "pussycat," "little sister," and "baby sister." This didn't bother me. I was happy Doren was writing to me at all and that her letters were affectionate.

———————

Dear Pussycat—

. . . Stop crying. Sleep, if you have to—but do a bit of work too—it's only for your own sanity to not fail. Anyway, it's almost summer and you can look forward to being a big-shot . . . at the ripe old age of 15 (Hey, I'll be 19 soon!!!! Eeek!)

MARK IS MEAN—just don't think about how *cute* he is and how *sexy*, etc.—just concentrate on the bad things—like his *immaturity* about girls, etc. Then maybe you can balance yourself out. If you let yourself dream, you'll work yourself into a *fit*. If you try to be a little calm though, *Fate* just *might* make him come back to you (I'm superstitious—but it's like taking a bath when you want a phone call—if you don't hang around waiting for things to happen, then they seem to happen on their *own*). Enough philosophy —you probably know it all already, little precocious devil that you are. . . .

You couldn't dissect the pig? Awwwwwwwwww! (as Peter would say) . . . (Ooops. I want to forget about him.)

I'm coming home (soon). Hold on!

XOX, Big Sister D

Hi Pussycat—

I don't have any classes on Thursdays . . . so I thought I'd do something nice for my little sister. This is a squeaky postcard—

squeeze it and it says hello in "pussycat talk." Luv—don't be sad
—Big D

_____

Two big events for me that year were when my mother,
father, and I visited Doren at Bryn Mawr, and later her first
visit home. Both were disastrous.

As we drove up a country road to Doren's dormitory, I was
immediately jealous. Weeping willows, vine-covered brick,
bright red fall leaves, young women wearing big wool sweaters
and carrying piles of books. I felt as if I had entered the free
world—the free world being, of course, any place to live that
wasn't home. I thought Doren was very lucky. I thought she
had escaped. She didn't feel the same. And her unhappiness
irritated our father. He, too, felt she was in an enchanted place
and saw no reason why she shouldn't have been thrilled.

_____

Today my parents and sister visited me for the first time. My
parents came bearing gifts and tokens of guilt. . . . My father almost wrecked my stereo when he inserted the new needle. We
had a screaming fight over that and finally my mother made him
leave the room so she could talk to me. . . .

"Doren, what's wrong with you? You look absolutely terrible.
What's wrong, darling?"

She kept asking me what was wrong and I chanted Nothing,
Nothing, until I couldn't take it anymore, so I told her I missed
New York and Peter and, for the second time in twelve hours, I
cried.

My father continued to inform me that I was very lucky to be in
such a fine college—and such a beautiful one—and when I
showed him the enormous, ivy-covered, neo-Gothic library, he
said in a choked voice, "I wish I could come here for a few
months. Just to read and think and be peaceful. I wish I could."
When I said I'd be glad to trade places with him he was, of course,
horrified by my ingratitude.

The worst part of the day was when they left. As I watched the
car pull away I suffered the pain of abandonment as if for the first
time.

_____

I was so busy imagining myself living at a place like Bryn
Mawr that I managed to avoid most of the day's tension. Or
rather, ignore it. I was filled with wonderful fantasies from the
visit and wrote to Doren as soon as I returned home.

Dear Doren—

I guess you know I think your college is beautiful—every part of it. I hope I'll be able to go to a college like it —if not Bryn Mawr itself. But let's face it—I'm not that smart. I just hope you don't get sick of me because I'll be popping up every once in a while. I'll be sure to bring an extra pillow when I come. . . .

Tell all your friends I thought they were great. Tell Elizabeth I can't wait to meet her, and tell Candice I thought she was really sweet and very pretty. I wish my "friends" were as nice as yours, Doren. . . .

The next time you speak to Peter or write to him, will you tell him that I say "Hi"?

Have a grand time and think of me battling the problems of life.

I Luv You, Big Sister

Dear Pussycat—

You are going to be a *terrific* girl very soon and be happy (relatively)—just wait and see. I never believed anyone when they told me that, but it's true. You have all the equipment you need— you're intelligent and sensitive and sharp and you're a real *Knockout* (everybody here thought you were a *beauty*) and you're much smarter than I am even about just getting along with people. You just have to be *philosophical* and think that if you put in lots of miserable time, you'll have to get *some* happy time, eventually. I really believe there is a symmetry to life—a balance—and after the total confusion of years 12–15, things start to balance out. You even get an idea of who you are and you even get to *like* it. . . . I know how frustrated you feel but *believe me,* this is the *worst* right now. I *PROMISE.*

. . . I love you very much and listen, if you ever want to visit— if you just *can't stand* being at home anymore—come to visit me. Even if I go out for a while, there's always some one of my friends who would keep you company—or else you could just enjoy my fabulous room alone. O.K.?

Elizabeth wants to meet you. Lisa thinks you're nice. Candice thinks you're just beautiful.

I love you, *baby sister*—Love, *big sister*

I visited Doren only once during the two years that she was at Bryn Mawr. The idea of being alone with my sister at her school felt good to fantasize about, but transforming the fantasy into reality was too frightening. As much as I wanted to escape the tensions at home, I was far too insecure to initiate leaving. Even temporarily.

The next family reunion, Doren's first visit, was another laugh a minute. This time the tension was between Doren and me.

The apartment was dark when I returned home that night. I concluded that Doren had arrived exhausted and that she had probably gone to sleep early. I was a bit crestfallen, more than a bit insulted. She could at least have waited up for me, I thought. I hadn't seen my sister in months and it was only in that moment I realized how much I had missed her.

I padded quietly down the hall, turned the knob on my bedroom door gently so it wouldn't squeak, and crept in. I could hear Doren breathing. I smiled at the familiar sound. On the way to my closet I bumped into something. I was startled. I had that room memorized. What could possibly crop up in the middle of my path to the closet? I reached down and felt the end of my bed. This was mystifying. My bed was not where it was supposed to be.

Once inside the closet I turned on the light and opened the door a crack to peek out. I experienced a fierce adrenaline rush. The room was not as I had left it.

From what I could see, it had been transformed, as closely as possible, minus the divider, back to the way it was before Doren had moved out. My shock turned to rage. I wanted to murder my sister. What I did was lock myself in the bathroom, sit on the closed toilet seat, and fume. I couldn't imagine how I'd ever pay her back for this intrusion. I couldn't imagine what had inspired such injustice and the rash assumption that she still had territorial rights in that room.

The battle that ensued involved some clawing. We both had big red welts on our arms to show for it. The room stayed that way while Doren was home, and I shifted everything back to my liking after she was gone.

Just because we were no longer living under the same roof didn't mean the power struggle had ended. Sibling rivalry dies hard. In truth, it dies not at all.

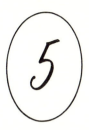

It is the three of us. Mother, Doren, and me. I am
fifteen. It is so hot the sea and sand merge into white.
This is Puerto Rico. I am being warned by my mother
and sister not to stay in the sun for very long ("The
sun is different here. . . .") and to cover my skin with
lotion. I love the sun and I despise lotion and the sun
doesn't feel any different to me. It is the first day of
our vacation. My parents have just separated. My
mother thought it would be a good idea if she treated
the three of us to a vacation. She felt it was a time we
should be together. For the remainder of the week,
Doren and I have purple skin from sun poisoning. We
lie still, in a bed we have to share, moaning in pain.
If our legs accidently touch, we yelp. The close prox-
imity is more than we can bear. Mother suggests
perhaps we cut our vacation short. We refuse to
leave on the grounds that perhaps we will heal before
long.

It is the three of us. Mother, George, and me. Mother
and George were recently married. I will be thirty in
two months. The sun is different here. Florida. Key
Biscayne. Palm trees. I walk miles down the beach
toward a lighthouse singing Joni Mitchell lyrics—"The
Minus is loveless/He talks to the land/And the leaves
fall/And the pond over-ices/She don't know the system, Plus/She don't understand/She's got all the
wrong fuses and splices/She's not going to fix it
up/Too easy. . . ." It has been one week since
Doren died. I am trying to find her. Wishing she
would find me. Asking her to. Mother and George
thought it would be a good idea if we went away
together. We are not away from anything. Lime-
green sea water. Dead Portuguese man-of-war
washed up on the beach, tentacles soaked and
matted. We do not have any notion that we will heal
before long.

I was fifteen when my parents separated. It was Doren's second year living away from home. That year I stopped pretending Mark would fall madly in love with me. Doren stopped pretending Peter would return from California. She began spending time with someone new, and brought him home over a holiday. My mother and I loved Reed. But Doren didn't seem happy.

I'm always nervous, self-conscious, and stiff. I find that instead of crying or writing or harboring secret fantasies of a better life to come, I frequently become rigid—by that I mean that I can't move. My arms and legs go numb about twice a day. In the middle of a class I am startled to discover I'm sitting on my hand or that I've been clutching a book so tightly there are ridges in my palms.

I swing back and forth between agonizing desire and the coldest apathy. In my apathetic state, like the narrator of Lessing's *The Golden Notebook,* I cannot believe I will ever feel desire again. . . . Sometimes I become so ashamed of my coldness that I attempt to be really kind to someone. . . .

Candice has become fearfully jealous of Reed because he takes up so much of my time. A recent (and typical) note: "What do you see in that arched back; that bright, wavy hair; those gleaming, swearing, piercing, dying ice-man eyes?"

I must confess that when Reed is angry the coldness of his eyes is terrible to behold (quite like Gerald in *Women in Love*). But he isn't cold by nature—just controlled.

Love is a word that never comes up in our conversations. . . .

My mother and I virtually adopted Reed. The timing was perfect—my father had just moved out and whether anyone was willing to confess it or not, the house became one filled with longing. Doren's relationship with Reed was an antidote for all of us. Although he and Doren did not visit frequently, he became the central man in all our lives. He was warm, gentle, sweet, amusing, and, most important, attentive. It seemed he needed to take care of us as much as we needed to be taken care of. Sometimes I felt Doren was happier about what Reed was doing for my mother and me than about her own relationship with him.

Reed is strange. Can't tell about him yet. Fear asking for anything—don't know what he thinks is too much. . . .

Reed is now a passion. Indispensable. Painful. Joyous. Warm.
Strengthening. But he doesn't love me yet. He's got to love me.
Reed has 1,000 obligations. I do not come first. Or even second a
lot of the time. . . . It pains me, but I think maybe sometime it will
happen. . . .

As unhappy as Doren was, it seemed to me she always
had her arm linked around that of a male, a male she could
refer to as "boyfriend." I wanted the same privilege. I wanted,
like Doren, to lead a "normal" life. I was tired of going to
dances with my girlfriends. Unfortunately, I had a habit of
ignoring any boy who dared to pay attention to me. I broke the
habit, temporarily, with Richie. He was persistent, and one
day I looked at him and thought, "Maybe I can have a boyfriend just like Doren always has."

Doren and I talked about Reed and Richie with each other,
and their names appeared frequently in our journal pages. The
fact that our father and mother separated received little verbal,
or written, attention. Only once did I give it notice, and Doren
not at all.

My parents separated—my father left today. . . . He
will be living across the street from his office. My mother
said they were both crying this morning. Every once in a
while I get a lump in my throat. . . . It's for the best—and
I'm mature.
School was lousy today. It also rained.

A few days later I put at the top of a page: "Maturity, Understanding, Pain." And that was that.

Except I began to fail every class I was in. The problem became so severe, my mother was called in. I knew that what
was being said behind my back was that my doing poorly in
school was a result of my parents' separation. I offered my
unsolicited opinion that this was sheer nonsense. I had more
important things to do—like going to parties, going out with
Richie, and being hired by school rock bands as a go-go dancer.

These were the days, the mid-sixties, when go-go dancing
had just come into popularity. Two girls dancing on either side

of a band, sometimes in boxes resembling small cages, was in. I became one of those dancers, thrilled I had finally found something I excelled in and Doren did not.

Doren, however, encouraged my dancing. She thought it was wonderful, and she saw how much I loved it. My mother was more concerned. She would see me when I came home late at night, my clothes disheveled and dirty, my hair matted, my body sweat-drenched, and I would always be grinning in ecstasy. She was not sure how to deal with my appearance and demeanor. Although I knew of her concern, she did not discourage me. In fact, she gave me advice on my wardrobe. She encouraged me not to wear the popular Courrèges white ankle boots that every other girl was wearing. She helped me pick out classy shoes and unusual, sophisticated outfits.

Dancing was the first thing in my life I *knew* I was good at. When I was ten years old, in fifth grade, I had won a trophy for best rock 'n' roll dancer. Ever since then Doren had been asking me to teach her steps. Then, when I became a go-go dancer at fifteen, my mother finally confessed she wished I would teach her a few things. I was determined to keep this ability to myself. I did not want my mother or Doren to know what I knew. I didn't want their feet copying mine. Although Mother would always chide me for not teaching her new steps, I never felt guilty.

My favorite pastimes the year my father moved out were doing as little schoolwork as possible, dancing and sweating as often as possible (the more sweat I produced, the happier I was —this desire would later come back to me in the form of running excessively and training for the New York Marathon when Doren was dying of cancer), and torturing Richie, inadvertently. He liked me a lot, and I was going to make him pay for it. My father was no longer living with my mother, and Richie got in the way of my misdirected rage. He was the first but not the last man in my life to become a target during a trying, lonely, and painful time for me, a time when I was experiencing loss.

One of the differences between Doren and me that had always been apparent was that I always had close female friends. Doren never formed the kind of friendships I did. Her associations with females were fleeting and fraught with competition. Doren confessed to me now and again that she did not trust women. She seemed to feel they wanted something from her, that she would be required to give pieces of herself away. Perhaps that is what she felt, for a long time, with me.

I, on the other hand, had an easier time trusting women than I did men. It seemed neither Doren nor I could sustain both intimate friendships with women and an intimate relationship with a man simultaneously. Doren always had a boyfriend and lacked the intimate woman friend. I always had nurturing relationships with girlfriends and lacked the intimacy with a man I wanted so much.

But, during my fifteenth year, and Doren's nineteenth, we both explored unfamiliar territory. I wanted to find a safe intimacy with a male whom I could also consider my friend. I found I could spend time with Richie in the same comfortable way I could with a girlfriend. The more at ease I became with our friendship, the more I entertained the notion of "going all the way." Doren was seeing Reed, but she was also beginning to explore the possibility of real friendship with a woman. Doren's friendship with Candice deepened. They admired each other, they respected each other's privacy, they laughed together, they confided in each other. It was a kind of closeness Doren had not allowed into her life before now.

Note from Candice:

Doren is my friend because

She is good
She worries
She has good taste
She dreams symbolically
She is funny
She thinks as I do
She eats a lot
and because
It is almost Christmas
and time to be happy.

Candice and I decided to play hooky today and go to the museum. As I might have expected, she wanted us to spend our time exclusively at the Greek pottery and artifacts section so she could impart to me her wealth of information on red and black figure painting. To me the only noteworthy thing about our pottery gazing was the inordinate number of gargantuan phalluses we were able to observe in just three hours.

After lunch I convinced Candice it would do her good to look at some French painting with me, and for a while we reversed roles as I swelled with nearly articulate admiration for Matisse, Picasso, Bonnard, Vuillard, etc. Meanwhile, Candice did her best not to look bored.

There was a little hall of contemporary sculpture, however, which provided by far the greatest pleasure of the afternoon. I discovered a 3½ foot Jean Arp in an obscure corner, and dared to touch the marble. Zounds! I brought Candice over to feel it; she had to suppress a cry of delight.

The exquisite cool marble was like some euphoric drug absorbed through the skin.

We took turns watching out for the guard, whose duty was to deprive us of the pleasure of touching, and for more than twenty minutes we shared an incredible sensual exaltation.

During the train ride back to school we didn't speak at all. Candice finally broke the silence at the dorm.

"If I ever met anyone with skin like that marble, I would be bound forever."

I nodded agreement.

It was almost five o'clock—still an hour and a half before dinner. It seemed unthinkable to mar the day with an attempt at work, so we lowered the shades in Candice's room, lit some incense and a candle in a big brass candlestick, dropped some records on the stereo, and lay back to dream.

Candice had smoked five cigarettes when she asked me with feigned nonchalance what I thought of Marnie.

I told her Marnie had made a pass at me in the shower and Candice laughed anxiously.

"Would you believe she did the same thing to me last week?"

"You're kidding."

"I was so uptight I wasn't going to tell you. She's weird, isn't she?"

"Mmmm."

"What do you think about it?"

"About what?"

"Making it with girls! What do you think?"

"Well, there are times when I feel horny enough to make it with animals, but I never seriously considered acting out any of my fantasies. . . ."

I paused while Candice watched me intently. "I told you how much I liked Cleo when we first became friends. . . . She was very undeveloped—androgynous in fact. . . . Well, we once started kissing at a party, but when we realized what was happening we had a long talk and decided that our attraction was just the intensity of new friendship and that we both still preferred the opposite sex."

Candice lit another cigarette.

"How about you?" I asked.

"Nothing, I guess. . . . Except you, sometimes."

"Me?"

"Does it make you uncomfortable? I don't intend to do anything about it."

I was silent.

"Does it turn you off?"

"No. I don't think so."

Candice took off the Rolling Stones and put on Tim Buckley. She draped herself across the bed, unconsciously, I suspect, imitating in her pose a suggestive photograph which her father keeps on his desk at home. She bent over to touch my hair. Then she sat down beside me on the floor.

"That sculpture was something else."

I nodded.

"I'll never forget it, will you?"

"Nope."

"Wow."

"Ummm."

Silence.

"You're uptight because of what I said, aren't you?" Candice asked.

"Why do you say that?"

"Because it's true."

"No, it isn't. I'm just thinking . . ."

"Mmmm."

She was touching my hair again, stroking it. It felt good. Then she rubbed my back for a while and that felt good too.

"Well?" Candice whispered.

"Well what?"

"Well, all I have to do is move my bureau up against the door and we're safe."

"Oh."

Candice moved her bureau up against the door, put some more records on, and sat down on the bed, and it was just like in the hall of pottery—she was the instructor and I was the student.

She reached for my head and pulled it close to hers to kiss my mouth.

Juicy, but un-erotic.

She seemed to reflect for a second, then brought her body on top of mine.

Her breasts rubbed heavily against my breasts; her groin felt heavy and bony. I tried to think sexy thoughts, but nothing happened.

I opened my eyes and noticed that it was 6:25. Soon a bustling crowd hungry for dinner would start growing outside Candice's room (which was just a few doors away from the dining room).

"Candice, it's time to eat."

"O.K."

When she sat up Candice looked decidedly glum.

"Are you turned on?" I asked timidly.

"I don't think so." Her mouth began a cautious, upward curve. "How about you? Anything?"

"Nope."

We looked straight into each other's eyes and burst out laughing.

Then we moved the bureau back and went to dinner, elbows linked.

My only fear about losing my virginity was that I would be doomed to love whoever accompanied me in that task for the rest of my life. This theory was fed to me by a girlfriend I considered reliable. I was not in the mood to love Richie forever, but I was definitely in the mood to lose my virginity.

The preparation for this event was so all-consuming that when it actually came to pass I was disappointed. More exciting had been the fact that I was keeping something this momentous in my life from my mother and sister. I consulted friends about where to go to get a diaphragm. I spent days trying to figure out the best place to hide it once I had it (that place was with my journal, of course—high up in my closet), I spent hours practicing how to use it, weeks feeling terrified the doctor I went to would find out I had given her a false name and was wearing a disguise (my hair up in a hat; dark glasses) and that she would call my mother and tell all, weeks being terrified that losing my virginity would be the most physically painful thing I would ever experience in my entire life (worse than my Puerto Rico sunburn) and that I would possibly bleed to death and then my mother and sister would find out what I had done. All this was so pressing I completely forgot about being worried that I might be compelled to love Richie for the rest of my life.

The memorable evening did not go exactly as planned. Richie and I had set our rendezvous for a night his parents and little sister would not be home. He took me out to a French restaurant, ordered wine, toasted us, had love in his eyes. This part was thrilling. Then we went to his house and we were greeted by his older sister, who had decided to come home from college on a surprise visit. We walked around the neighborhood for hours, waiting for her to go out with her boyfriend. Eventually she did leave. We went back upstairs, and while I struggled in the bathroom with an uncooperative diaphragm, Richie prepared his bedroom. This preparation consisted of changing the sheets to old ones he could throw away after we were through with them, and when I emerged from the bathroom into a pitch-dark room, I had to help him shove his bureau up against the bedroom door—just in case. He put on a Mamas and Papas album, playing "Dedicated to the One I Love" over and over again, and as we were nervously getting to it, the phone rang. Richie had forgotten he had to pick up his little sister from her dance class. We got dressed, rearranged the room, changed the sheets back, walked with wobbly knees to pick up his sister, returned to the house to find that now his older sister was home again, decided we were going to go ahead with this anyway, retreated into his bedroom, changed the room again, played the Mamas and Papas again. I kept a pillow squeezed over my face in case I screamed with pain, and, in a remote manner of speaking, we made love.

Later, when Richie was putting me into a taxi and I was noticing how he had forgotten to put his socks back on before putting on his penny loafers, I asked him if he felt any different about me now and he said that now he loved me more. I did not say the same to him.

_____

Sometimes I damn the day I decided to consider the male race as a source of pleasure, and sometimes I fantasize a love who could be skin-close in no time at all, and a place to be alone with him, and a car to take us wherever we want to go. . . .

The root of the problem has appeared for some time to be sex, and it vexes me greatly to admit it. The fact that I need to define myself as a woman, and can't seem to do it independently. I would like not to need a man. I would like to be a human hermaphrodite, sufficient unto myself. Then I would be capable of intimate friendships with men or women without the inevitable hostilities generated by the demands of sexuality and the subsequent battles for dominion. . . .

. . . I sit in my little dormitory room in the semidarkness and stare out the window at the air, or move aimlessly from my bed to my desk chair, and it's like being a piece of dust—I seem to have lost myself—mind, body—everything.

I talked to Candice about this feeling and she said my sickness is the result of believing in the potential union of mind and body. She said it's a common human failing, but that I should be clever enough to know that the desire for oneness is a death wish, and that happiness will come only when I stop trying to pull myself into an integrated whole and accept the dichotomy—and the subsequent multiplicity of personality—for what it is—permanent and irreversible. She says she has done this, and she's never been happier or more relaxed. In other words, she's relinquished everything to the pleasures of the flesh, and since she's screwing Jonah several times daily, she has little time for mental anguish. . . .

I didn't feel any different about Richie after losing my virginity, but I did feel different about me. I felt as though I were a part of the world, now that I had been let in on the big secret. I remember sitting on a Central Park West bus the next day, heading downtown, wondering if anyone could tell just by looking at my face. I felt different, so I supposed I looked different too. I was sure that part of the child had fallen away and the look of a woman had replaced it.

By this time my mother was frequently out in the evenings. Many of her social engagements were related to her job as a publicist. I didn't like it. Not at all. I especially resented her not always returning home at the time she had told me she would. Of course I forced her to give me an exact time when I could expect her return. She would do this to appease me, to thwart my hassling her more than I already was. I spent many nights curled into the butterfly chair in my bedroom, shivering even if it wasn't cold, watching Johnny Carson, listening to all the creaks and clicks and sighs and groans of the apartment walls and floors, praying I would hear the sound of the elevator and my mother's key in the door because—just as I had been years before in Merrick, waiting for my parents to return home at night—I was terrified. But now it was different. Now I didn't have Doren. My sister was out there, somewhere, but the physical comfort of her was no longer with me.

I would be turning sixteen soon and I wanted to do what all the other girls I knew were doing. I wanted to have a Sweet Sixteen. All my girlfriends were having Sweet Sixteen parties at fancy hotels. My choice was the Copacabana, where The Supremes would be performing around the time of my birthday.

My invitation list was curious indeed. It included every boy I had ever had a crush on. Richie was not pleased. I tried to persuade him that what I was doing was quite harmless, and the only control he achieved was over the seating arrangements. He told me he'd kick Mark incessantly if I sat them across the table from each other. No harm came to anyone that night and I couldn't have been happier being the center of attention.

After my birthday came mononucleosis, a.k.a. The Kissing Disease. I held Richie responsible for my misfortune, and no longer wanted to be with him. Everyone teased me. Even Doren. She had come home to visit and informed me that now she knew Richie and I had been doing a lot of kissing. I was so angry I informed *her* this wasn't all we had been doing. She was startled—then, as I lay in bed for weeks with a high fever, Doren completely ignored me. She refused to help take care of me. She would not be tied down. She would not believe I was as sick as I was. She was as angry as she had been when I had first gotten my period. I was no longer a virgin. Another shift. I was catching up with her.

I just can't imagine a life completely wrapped around a man and a house. I need to feel the significance of my *own* life—it seems to me that to be a wife and mother in the everyday functions these titles require is to be merely a kind of servant. . . .

I fear an early marriage would be deadlier to me than a fatal disease. . . . I begin to understand the compulsion to bear children regardless of the factors of husband (or lover), practical consideration (age, school), etc.

For the last few weeks Candice has been moody and short-tempered and tonight she finally offered an explanation. She entered my room with an apology for her recent bitchy behavior and a dramatic announcement:

"I am pregnant."

. . . I'll go home with her next weekend to help her get through the birthday celebration her parents have planned for her. Candice refuses to tell her parents; she claims it would destroy them, and further, that they would probably forbid her to have an abortion. . . .

Candice's farm is lovely and sad and solemnly autumnal. . . .

We eat from heavy pewter dishes that belonged to her mother's great-grandmother. Wine is served with lunch and dinner, and from late spring to late fall there are home-grown fruits and vegetables—onions, beans, corn, four kinds of lettuce, tomatoes the size of melons, melons as large as small pumpkins, etc.

There is little furniture in the house, but all of it has been made by Candice's father, who taught himself carpentry about ten years ago when the barn was wrecked by a hurricane. Determined to find a constructive use for the remains of the barn, he learned how to build furniture.

Candice's parents have never owned a television set, but they've recently installed quite a good stereo, which fills the living room with Bach, Mozart, Vivaldi, and Couperin after dinner.

Today is Candice's eighteenth birthday. From her father she received two watercolors (his own) and a beautiful wooden record chest with brass fittings which he made himself. From her mother she received an Irish fisherman sweater and a suede belt from Germany.

The little party was difficult for Candice because her parents reminisced quite a lot about her childhood and old times. Her father got out a book he made for her when she was very small entitled *Candice in the Forest*. He had illustrated and bound it, and her mother had written the text.

The pictures of the blond little girl and her animal friends were inexpressibly poignant. What a picturesque childhood Candice must have had on the farm. For a split second I was jealous of her, but then I remembered her present sorrow and repented. . . .

We talked about growing up. I had to agree that Candice's transition had been more difficult than mine—that is, if such a thing is measurable.

One day when she was twelve—after her breasts had become quite large—she found a bra in the underwear drawer of her dresser, placed there furtively by her mother. She was happy not to have had to ask for it—she would have been too embarrassed to ask—but upon trying it on discovered it was far too small. She spent the rest of the day locked in her bathroom, sewing on two pieces of cloth from the rag box—to make the bra wider around the back. And she wore it every day for two years. . . .

Candice's abortion will be tomorrow. . . . I quiet my own fears by remembering that the "abortionist" is, after all, a doctor who will not cause her permanent injury. . . .

It's 12:45 A.M. and Candice has just returned. She looks gray and informs me she is still bleeding at the rate of three napkins per hour.

I bring her some food I saved from dinner and make her eat a little of it.

She falls asleep in a state of delirium, mumbling something incoherent about her "son."

I don't want to leave her alone, so I'll get some blankets from my room and sleep on her floor.

I find it difficult to believe, but she claims she was given no anesthetic whatsoever prior to surgery.

"My son, my son . . . Would I have died for thee." The words plagued her as she lay in her narrow bed, trying to sleep. . . .

The clock in the doctor's office. Watching it upside down and closing her eyes and then opening them again, thinking she had fainted. And what time was it now? Was it over?

The doctor whispering, "You must be quiet. . . . Remember, you must be quiet. . . ."

And the water pouring out of the cold-water tap across the room—"In case the office is bugged," he had explained.

And looking at the clock upside down. Trying to concentrate on the numbers of the clock.

Whispering, "9:30 upside down means it's really . . . really what? 9:30 upside down means . . . 3:00 . . . 3 o'clock. . . ."

Sliding in and out of consciousness . . .

And, finally, the doctor telling her to put on her "panties." Giving her a few pain pills for "later." Asking her to hurry so he can start on his next "customer."

And the doctor kissing her on the mouth. Hard on the mouth.

She closed her eyes and at once the image of the doctor's office returned. She surveyed the office with the meticulousness of a detective.

Where did he put it when he took it out of her? Where, god-damnit?

"Where did he put my son?"

———————

Doren, who had always wanted a child, she said, for as long as she could remember, dreaded abortion. She knew she would have an abortion if the circumstances were not right for having a child, if they were not in the child's best interest, but she prayed such circumstances would never arise. "Where are my children going to come from?" she'd say wistfully from time to time, wondering who their father would be. When Doren considered a relationship with a man, she would consider in the first moments of infatuation whether or not she could imagine that man as the father of her children. This was as important as imagining whether or not this man could be her lover.

Just prior to Doren discovering she had cancer, she discovered she was pregnant. The man she had been involved with for years did not feel ready to have a child. Doren did not want her child to be without a father. And she was not in a position in her life to be able to raise a child on her own. After careful, painful hours of consideration, Doren had an abortion. She was still in disbelief that she had lost her first child when she was, just months later, faced with the possibility of losing her own life. Doctors informed her that if she had sustained her pregnancy, the cancer would most likely have spread like wildfire. This was no consolation to her. Doren's sorrow over her abortion stayed with her, huge and silent.

During the summer of 1967, Doren, unhappily, went off to Cambridge, Massachusetts. Reed had told her he wanted some "space." So Doren decided to go to Harvard summer school. Perhaps the new environment would lessen the pain of separation. I went off that same summer to Trebor for the last time. It was there that I could write out in the open, sing, dance, act, and have a heyday indulging in my creative resources without fear of comparison and feelings of inferiority. At Trebor I was always encouraged, my talents always acknowledged. Once in that environment, I lost all interest in what I considered to be the frivolous aspects of my life. Richie was one such frivolous aspect. Unfortunately, I thought the only creative, soulful people existed on this small lake surrounded by mountains in this remote high corner of northern Maine. This was where my true life was.

By the fall, Doren informed us she had met the man she was going to marry. He was doing post-doctoral work in physics at Harvard. She would transfer from Bryn Mawr to Barnard in New York, would get her own apartment, and would graduate from school early so that in December of the following year she and Andrew could marry.

She threw my mother, father, and me into a panic. Me because I automatically despised anyone who would dare to take Reed's place; my father because he was concerned about finances and did not want to subsidize her apartment or have to support her after she was married; my mother because she sensed disaster if Doren married at age twenty. On no count would Doren be swayed. She was convinced—this was *it*. And she was fully confident that after we all met Andrew we all would be convinced as well. The challenge was on.

Letter from Candice:

Marriage now is not for you because it is far from great. And it doesn't solve nobody's problems. Unfortunately. I started taking pills again this month and ended bleeding violently and clotting and having horrible pains for eight days. So I went to the gynecologist. Now I am off pills, I'm bleeding like hell, I have terrible pains. Last night I couldn't go to sleep even one time. Last night Rachel tried to kill herself, chickened out, cut herself all up instead. She was screaming so loudly that the whole dorm was running around moaning, "What has happened?" I went to Haverford and got drunk. . . . Sally's father was killed in a plane crash about two weeks ago. I want to come and see you but I can hardly move. . . . My current philosophy centers around hate: life, love, everybody, school, my room. . . . I cry a lot. Do you? Please write to me. . . .

Candice, my friend, my long-lost friend, why are you *bleeding?* If the gynecologist you go to isn't inspiring your confidence, *please* come to N.Y. and see mine. He's a very fine doctor and a very, very kind man. I'll even make the appointment for you if you want. Please let me know. And please, *please* come to visit me soon. I miss you very much and I think we need each other.

To speak of happier things . . . I am in love—truly in love. I'd love to tell you all the things I feel but they seem to come out as tired clichés. I'd love you to meet Andrew, though. Then you would understand. . . . Of course I miss him terribly when I'm in N.Y., but I've been seeing him often and when we're together it's so *good* and so *beautiful* and so *exciting* that it really does make up for the lonely times. Which is not to say that we're always "happy" together—but that we are growing more and more together all the time. . . . Believe it or not, *he's* the one who's been talking about marriage. I try not to say too much because I want him to think about it on his own. As for me, I am absolutely certain I want to spend my life with him—if it's possible—and I want to have *his* children. . . .

Do you think I'm crazy? The only thing that scares me is thinking that something might happen to Andrew, or me, and then we couldn't be together. . . .

Don't ever think you don't have a friend. I'm here and I'm for you.

Letter from Candice:

. . . I knew before I asked you for your news that you are in love again—or is it really again and not maybe the first real time? . . . But what happens to Reed?

. . . I really miss you and sing of woe. . . . Would you like to go to the Metropolitan with me one day soon and see Greek vases and sculpture? . . . I want to come and see you, my friend. . . .

Dear Candice—

. . . Andrew has asked me to marry him—not for the first time, but for the first time *seriously*. Yesterday when we were eating breakfast. And when he finished (proposing?) he burped (my coffee). Of course I only half-believe him, but it seems more possible all the time. We had an all-night talk—fight—I don't know *what*—Saturday night—started by me in desperation. I have been feeling absolutely miserable because I have to work like a dog all week to get enough stuff done to come here (e.g., a paper due every Monday at 3:00), and then I have to lug myself here—almost 5 hours each way by car (I've been getting rides to save money)—each weekend. It's pretty much of a drain. So I wanted to let Andrew know that this situation is taking its toll on me, but all weekend I felt too guilty to burden him with it—I know *he* can't come to see *me* because he has research and teaching and school (classes) responsibilities (even on Saturdays) and so I can't condemn him for putting the burden of traveling on me. But I finally blurted out my misery—in typical whining fashion—and when he insisted on going to sleep, I insisted on a fight. God it was awful. It wasn't even a screaming fight—just cold-blooded talking and "logic," which makes the whole universe blacker by the minute. By 4:30 A.M. suicide was beginning to look like the only answer. And then somehow the tide turned. I don't know why, but we just never seem to be able to be estranged from each other for too long. Everything fell away. Especially logic. And we were reconciled. It all had the effect of a long separation (in time) on the two of us. And it has changed our relationship in a very positive way. There seems to be something more solid between us now. . . . And marriage—I don't know. I feel I must finish school before I do (get married) and I suppose Andrew does too. So I am going to submit a petition at Barnard to graduate in February 1969—a semester early. And Andrew wants to marry me then. Does it sound real to you? I guess not, but I'm beginning to believe in it. . . .

. . . Unless we see each other soon we might as well stop writing because I trust words on paper less all the time, and I know that letters are not preventing us from becoming absolutely out of touch with each other. So please try to come sometime. . . .

I cried profusely, as if it were me and not Reed that Doren was breaking up with. No one, I thought, could possibly be as wonderful as Reed. Doren grew increasingly enraged as I kept locking myself in the bathroom sobbing and yelling, "How can you do this? How can you do this to Reed?" I don't think the separation I was most concerned about was the one between Doren and Reed. Where would my relationship with Doren be once she had a husband?

I was home the night Doren had planned to break the news to our beloved Reed. When he arrived Doren led him into the dining room and closed the door. She had instructed me not to come out and greet him but she promised she would tell him I wanted to see him before he left. I sat in the kitchen eating cold cereal. It was early evening. I had no appetite and I couldn't stop crying, and when I pulled a prize out of the cereal box and it was an orange dinosaur I thought it a good omen because Reed had orange-red hair. I didn't know anything about Zen at the time, but I was concentrating awfully hard on transmitting messages to Reed in the dining room—talk her out of it, talk her out of it, talk her out of it. . . .

Their meeting was brief. I heard Reed walking quietly across the front hallway floor and then I heard the front door shut. He left without saying a word to me. He had adopted me and now I felt like an abandoned child. Again.

I wouldn't let Doren off the hook. I screamed and yelled and cried more than she did. She pleaded with our mother to get me off her case. "I don't understand why you're so upset!" Doren yelled at me. "He wasn't *your* boyfriend, for chrissake!"

As she had done with Paul McCartney, Doren set out to convince me that Andrew was "the cuter Beatle," the better boyfriend-soon-to-be-husband. I was not about to betray Reed. He told Doren that he had not intended for their relationship to end. He had, in fact, returned from the summer wanting to more seriously commit himself to Doren. But it was too late.

Determined to bring me over to her side, Doren took me into her confidence and described how she and Andrew had met. It was a love-at-first-sight story and, being sixteen, it was hard for me not to be seduced by it.

Doren had been having an unhappy summer in Cambridge. She was angry at Reed for suggesting a separation she did not feel was mutual. She did the only thing she knew how to do under these circumstances—she threw herself into her work at Harvard summer school. Socializing was out of the question. She did not want to subject anyone to her poor frame of mind.

One evening a few women who lived in the apartment above hers were having a party. They were women who were always trying to befriend Doren, but Doren felt she had nothing in common with them. On this night one of them came downstairs and knocked on Doren's door to inform her they were having a party and that she was invited.

Doren sat on her bed for hours, pondering the issue. She was in no mood to be around any human being, let alone many at a party. She felt rotten, she looked in the mirror and decided she also looked rotten. Her hair was dirty and she had a very large pimple on the tip of her nose. This was definitely not a party face. The alternative to going was feeling sorry for herself, and Doren remembered the words our mother would always say to us—"You never know!" Doren knew that, if consulted, my mother would advise her to go. Why stay home when clearly nothing good could come of that? But, if the choice were made to venture out—You never know!

Doren did not want to go as far as to wash her hair—she had already expended enough energy deciding to go to the party. She put her hair up with a rubber band in a high ponytail right at the top of her head, "like Pebbles Flintstone" she told me. She spent about twenty minutes struggling to camouflage the prominent pimple with her cover-up stick but this was a futile task. She didn't want to dress up, given that it was a hot and sticky night, so she wore what she already had on—a little summer dress that made her look twelve years old. As Doren walked out the door she said to herself, "This one's for you, Ma."

When she walked into the party the first face Doren saw was Andrew's. He was at the other end of the room, and Doren said he moved toward her grinning widely. She was immediately charmed and flattered. Andrew walked straight over to her and the first thing he did was wipe the makeup off her nose she had spent all that time trying to perfect. She excused herself, found the bathroom, reapplied the makeup to her pimple, and returned to Andrew.

Birth of a marriage. They were together for the rest of the evening and through to the following morning. Never mind that months later Andrew confessed he had been very high on that fateful evening and that when Doren walked in he thought she was someone else, someone he knew and hadn't seen in a long time. Also, in his condition, he became fascinated with the pimple on her nose and couldn't understand why she kept covering it up. He did say he loved her dress right off the bat, especially later when he discovered it could slip off Doren's body all in one motion—no buttons, no snaps, no zippers, no fumbling. Apart from all that, his feeling of love for Doren that night (he reassured her) was most definitely authentic.

Doren was more nervous about bringing Andrew home than I was. The stakes were high, and my approval meant more to Doren than it ever had before. She knew it would be foolish to trust our parents to be objective, but for some reason she felt it was wise to trust that I would be. Under the circumstances, it would have been more appropriate for Andrew to ask me for Doren's hand in marriage than to ask my father. My father insisted he wanted that gesture extended to him. Doren argued briefly about this, then obliged him reluctantly. She thought he was behaving in an archaic manner.

———

Dear Candice—

Yes, I am *really* engaged. *Really engaged.* I've been working so hard the last few weeks I haven't even had a chance to remember how happy and excited I am about it.

When will I ever see you again? I'm leaving tomorrow for Cambridge. . . . I'm really sorry I have to turn down your offer to come to N.Y. *I really miss you!* I think I'm having a small engagement party (my mother wants to do it for me) the first week in April. I'll be on vacation—will you? I'll be desolate if you can't come, so if you tell me now you can't I'll change the date. . . . Please let me know. But I want to see you before then, of course. And I'm dying for you and Andrew to meet. Not that I have any doubts I'm doing the right thing—but I would really be happy if you like him too.

I'm submitting a petition at Barnard to graduate early—next January instead of June (1969) and the minute I graduate—or soon after—I hope Andrew and I will get married. . . .

How are your parents? I'd really love to visit them again—there is such a good *peace* at your house.

I MISS YOU
I'M SICK OF STUDYING
I'M TIRED OF COLD WEATHER
   -BUT-
I'M MADLY IN LOVE

and somehow I'm going to survive college so I can have my life. . . .

Enter Andrew. Handsome, warm, funny, humble, with a face so similar to Doren's it was uncanny. Presto. He was family. He was someone I could easily adore. He was kin. The immediate familial aura was so pronounced that one day Doren slipped and called out to Andrew in another room— "Mommy!" Everyone's laughter did little to assuage the moment of shock and utter bewilderment we all experienced from the most potent Freudian slip we had ever heard. Years later, when Doren was married to Andrew, she expressed her feeling more directly.

To Cathy last night on the phone (re Andrew and my mother):
"I think of them both in much the same way."
And then I start to giggle and, literally, blush and I tell C I have to hang up because I'm so embarrassed and C, laughing hysterically, too, still has the sensitivity to yell through hilarity, "You're not a freak. Don't think you're a freak!"

Dear Candice—

. . . You have to promise to come to the wedding no-matter-*what* because you're my only true friend and I really want you to be there. . . .

Letter from Candice:

. . . please forgive me if I do not come to your engagement party. Please don't be mad at me—and please let me come to see you soon. . . .

Dear Candice—

I didn't get your letter until Monday, so of course I waited and waited for your appearance at my party on Saturday night. I was very sad you didn't come, although I was sure you'd have a good reason, and Andrew was even more disappointed than I was. I know how clutched you must be about school, but, of course, I wish you had come for a few hours anyway. (I know you're not working *every single* minute—or are you?)

. . . The dinner with Andrew's family was really very pleasant —no fireworks whatsoever. And Andrew's sister asked me to be a bridesmaid at her wedding. I think that's a nice gesture. *And* his parents wanted some of my engagement pictures! I don't understand this whole business—my father and Andrew talked in absolute isolation for *two hours* (and when I listened in I heard only my *father's* voice).

Write—write—write.

————————

So I decided Andrew was no villain. I decided something far worse. I decided he was perfect.

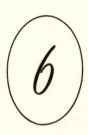

Doren's wedding. We are facing the rabbi. Doren is
wearing a white Mexican wedding dress, I am wearing
blue velvet. I am on one side of her, Andrew is on the
other. I am afraid to look at my sister. It is all I can do
to control myself from losing it completely and breaking out into loud sobbing. I can see Doren out of the
corner of my eye. Her face is so white, her chest is red
and getting redder; her infamous nervous bright red
rash is spreading out across her chest rapidly. I turn
my head slightly and we look right at each other. She
is having as much trouble as I am. I breathe deeply,
holding my breath, and she does the same. Any minute now we are both going to collapse into some form
of hysteria. I see Andrew trying to get Doren's attention, trying to get her to look at him as the rabbi is
speaking. She's resisting his coaxing. She is staring
straight ahead, concentrating very hard on remaining
upright.

Doren's service. A different rabbi. I am sitting on an
aisle seat, my mother is next to me, our hands are
locked together. The rabbi calls my name. It takes all
of the energy in my body to disengage my hand, rise
from my seat, slowly, very slowly, walk carefully to
the podium, turn to face the auditorium filled with
expectant, sad faces. I read two poems—one of Doren's, one of mine. I am not sure whose voice is emerging from my mouth, Doren's voice or my own. But
there is one thing I am sure of. She is up there with
me. She is making me strong. She is giving me the
confidence to proceed.

*D*oren returned to New York my junior year of high
school for her junior year of college. She had transferred to
Barnard and had convinced our father to help her out financially with her own apartment. My excitement about Doren

having an apartment in New York was as intense as if it was to
be my own. I spent many hours with her there, sitting at her
white bistro table, sipping tea with the steam heat hissing as
we talked, or propped up on pillows on her double bed as she
read me letters from her fiancé and we both grinned madly,
while listening to the radio waiting for our favorite songs to be
played. When I could not make out the words Doren would
de-code them for me. And when Andrew visited on weekends,
on breaks from his work at Harvard, I would accompany them
to museums, for walks in the park through snow, for pancakes
in or pancakes out early on Sunday mornings. With Doren and
Andrew I was content. I was happy. I was safe. My sister was
back.

I became increasingly disenchanted with the group of people
I had been spending time with for the past couple of years.
Outside of Doren and Andrew, I was bored. I began to make
some weekend trips to Boston to visit my camp friends there.
During one of those weekends I met the first young man I felt
I loved. Christopher approached me at a party, he knew my
name, I recognized him from my friend Joan's class at school
where I had visited previously, he sat down on the floor in
front of me, and I began to tremble. I was experiencing someone's total and complete concentration on me and on me alone.
I was flattered. I was terrified. I was suspicious.

———————

Dear Candice—

Cathy (my sister) is in love. She met some boy (16 years old) in
Boston a few weeks ago with *very* long hair and poetry in his soul.
I don't know what to think of the two of them—I know that it's
probably a fleeting thing, but I remember when I was sixteen and
how sure I felt about things and how intense and stubborn I was.
It makes me sad that their love probably won't last *forever*—but
who knows, maybe it will last a long time. People change so much
from 16–20 that one love seems impossible, but sometimes it
seems one love is impossible from 20 on as well. *Change is life*—
the problem is how to change and still be heading in the same
direction as the one you love. That's the problem. . . .

———————

Now Doren and I both had our respective men in Boston to
visit. What a coincidence. Doren would put signs up on the
bulletin boards at Barnard and Columbia for rides to and from

Boston and the two of us would drive up with various students on frequent Friday evenings. Christopher lived at home, so we needed a place "to be alone together." When Andrew and Doren were not at Andrew's apartment, they supplied us with that place. Once again, Doren was my ally.

Christopher hawked an underground newspaper in Boston, and if he sold enough papers after school during the week, he would have enough money to visit me in New York on the weekend. We faced the same problem in New York regarding privacy. Doren made a suggestion. Her former boyfriend Reed now had a new girlfriend and was frequently staying at her house—why didn't I call Reed and ask him if Christopher could stay at his apartment over a weekend? Reed was terribly kind and accommodating to both of us, and, I noticed, terribly nervous in my presence. Although Reed and Doren were now attempting a platonic relationship, I felt he was still in love with her. Apparently Candice thought the same.

Letter from Candice:

. . . Reed visited here this weekend and talked to me with sadness in his eyes and drawn wan cheeks for you, whom he loves yet. We had a sort of forced conversation for $2^1/_2$ minutes. Then he left. . . .

Whenever I spent time with Christopher, whether it was in Boston or in New York, I did not want to share that time with anyone else. Even if Doren and Andrew were also around, I did not instigate a foursome. I wanted to keep the threesome —Doren, Andrew, and me—intact. It was a configuration I did not want to tamper with, a safe balance.

I was not spending a great deal of time at home with my mother. Any man she would bring home, although no one ever spent the night, I felt was an intruder. She, in kind, was not at all pleased about Christopher. She had not known I had lost my virginity with Richie, and so she assumed Christopher was the culprit. She seemed to know we were sleeping together. For a while, every time she looked at me, she clicked her tongue in sorrow and defeat. She made it clear that she felt I was too young for the emotional ramifications that accompanied intimacy with a man. I thought, simply, that she did not know what she was talking about.

Christopher and I became involved in political protests and marches. Because my school was "progressive," the classes shifted their focus to accommodate the current political atmosphere. I cried with Christopher when Robert Kennedy and Martin Luther King were assassinated. He marched with me in New York; I marched with him in Boston.

I became angry at Doren that she was not as "politically active" as I was. Yet every time I had any question about current events, Doren could supply me the answer. She was my secret history teacher and always remained so. But the fact that she wasn't out marching annoyed me. Her time was spent either with Andrew or doing schoolwork. She was planning to graduate early so she could marry Andrew and move to Cambridge while he continued his post-doctoral work at Harvard.

During the summer of 1968 Doren went off to Cambridge to live with Andrew (in the fall she would move all her belongings as well), and Christopher came to New York to be with me. We were both seventeen and we wanted to live together, but, living at home, I was still under parental jurisdiction and I knew my mother would never allow it. Christopher managed to sublet an apartment in Washington Heights where I would go to be with him every night. Of course I would have to return home at a reasonable hour, and I remember the summer as a series of cab rides, staring out at the Hudson River as the cab whizzed by, the warm wind through the open window in my face, feeling sorry for myself that I was not allowed to spend the entire night with my loved one.

Christopher was working during the day in a bills-of-lading department at a shipping company, a job my mother helped him find through a friend. I was enrolled in acting classes at the Stella Adler Theater Studio. My journal stopped. It had stopped the moment I met Christopher. Doren's journal stopped as well. It stopped from the moment she met Andrew. The infamous dilemma—how-to-write-and-have-a-relationship-at-the-same-time—apparently began for both of us simultaneously. Our journals resumed later on, but only when we began having difficulty in our respective relationships.

Even though Christopher was in New York, I was unhappy. Most of the time I felt as sad as if I were completely alone. I went to acting classes during the day and saw Christopher when he got off work. I was lethargic. Doren and I were in minimal contact. She seemed so far away now.

By the end of the summer Christopher and I had started fighting. Even so, when the time came for him to return to

Boston, I fell apart, crying hysterically for days before he left, and weeks after he was gone. His departure felt like every abandonment I had ever experienced rolled up into one. I wasn't just unhappy, I was frightened. Missing Christopher was a label for my fear.

Dear Candice—

I really miss you! Andrew and I have been very busy moving. . . . The place was filthy and I've been scrubbing all week but now it looks quite good—we got a dresser for $5 and spent one day painting it a shiny enamel blue. Now we're trying to get the landlord to paint the apartment since it probably hasn't been painted for about 10 years. Soon it's bound to be a showplace, though. We've been doing all kinds of neat things, since in an unfurnished apartment you really start from scratch. . . .

How's your head? Smooth, prickly, or full of cheese and wine? If you read more than 10 books before you get back to school I'll be too much in awe of you to be your friend anymore, so *watch it!*

I'm not going to say anything about the Democratic National Convention because I'm just too upset. It was a nightmare.

. . . Please write to me and let me know what's happening to *you.* I'm sad that we're back to letters again but it's better than silence, right? . . .

Doren was to be married in December of 1968. There must have been a lot of preparation, yet I remember little if any of it. I kept myself apart from wedding activity. There was no way to compete with this event so I made myself scarce. The moderate-size wedding was to be held at a Central Park South hotel. I was excited for Doren, I thought Andrew was wonderful, I didn't agree with my parents that Doren was too young to be married, and I was jealous. Now, from the perspective of over thirty, I am stunned that Doren married when she was twenty . . . and divorced when she was twenty-four. I always thought she was as mature as a person old enough to be my parent. And she always imagined the same.

Dear Candice—

My life is completely up in the air at this minute. It looks like my wedding will have to be during Christmas vacation (either

December 21 or December 28) because the first weekend of intersession Andrew's father will be on a business trip, and the second weekend is too late because Andrew has to be back at school on Sunday, February 2. . . .

So keep December 21 and December 28 open. I'm pretty sure it's going to be one or the other. . . .

. . . You have to promise to come no-matter-*what* because you're my only true friend and I really want you to be there.

Letter from Candice:

OF COURSE I WILL COME TO YOUR WEDDING. What's it going to be like?

————————

During that fall I became less interested in sustaining a relationship with Christopher and more interested in school. I developed two priorities during my last year of high school—my Russian literature course and an infatuation with a math teacher, Kevin, whose class I was not taking. I began seeing Christopher less. I was reading one hundred pages a day of *Anna Karenina* while trying to figure out how to get close to Kevin. Being a senior, and given the flexible Walden rules, I managed to frequently get myself invited into the Teachers' Room. There was a teacher who was also attracted to Kevin. I knew she was, and she knew I was, and so we didn't like each other. As time went on, the entire high school knew of this "triangle." School kept me very busy and constantly titillated. A new phenomenon. Doren had been away from Walden long enough so that I felt I was no longer competing with her ghost. I could excel at school in my own right; I could be a big shot with the teachers; I could experience unabashed academic enthusiasm. I marked up *Notes from Underground* with so many exclamation points and shouts of "Yes!" you could barely read Dostoevsky's words.

How did I manage to develop an attraction to someone who was connected to Andrew? As it turned out, Kevin and Andrew had attended Cornell together as undergraduates. Did this discourage my infatuation for Kevin? No. *Au contraire.* All I needed to hear was that Andrew said Kevin was a nice guy and suddenly Kevin was not only appealing, he was legitimate. This was the beginning of a pattern. Most of the men I began to gravitate toward had some connection to either my sister or my mother. Doren often tried to get me to acknowledge the folly of my ways.

A couple of weeks before Doren's wedding my mother took me on a jaunt through the jewelry district. Doren's wedding ring had already been bought. I didn't understand why we were going shopping for jewelry. My mother had something unusual in mind. She was intent on buying me something, specifically a ring. Although I never questioned the gesture, I was vaguely aware of what she was doing—my mother didn't want me to feel left out. I picked out a beautiful antique ring. Sixteen years later, I am still wearing it. It did just what she had intended it to do. It made me feel special too.

At Doren's wedding I was not simply the maid of honor, but in some deep emotional sense it was as if I were being married with them, to them. Within two months of their marriage I was considering colleges only in Boston. I was back on track with Christopher. He was my reason for wanting to be in Boston. Or so I thought. Doren and Andrew would soon be taking care of their first child—me.

The newlyweds spent their honeymoon in New York, staying at a hotel and going to concerts and shows. I was busy that week as well—going to concerts and shows with the newlyweds. This was a marriage divinely conceived, I thought, and so it would never end. I had a fierce investment in my sister's marriage "working." This marriage was to be my role model. If it failed, I would never believe in relationships or marriage again.

Dear Candice—

I love you.

Andrew loves you (and won't stop reminding me how much fun it will be to visit you in Virginia and then camp out in the Smokies).

Dear Candice—

You might be moving to North Carolina, Oregon, Pennsylvania??? But if you go far away I'll never see you and you are my best friend. What will I do? Of course I have Andrew but even if he is my friend—which he is—he's a man and that's a whole other thing. . . . I haven't found anyone of our troubled sex that I could really depend on in the fullest sense of friendship—except for you. . . .

Dear Candice—

. . . IMPORTANT—I appreciate the fact that you now address your letters to both Andrew and me, but I feel concerned that this enlarged audience will cause you to alter the content of your letters. If I am right, then please go back to addressing letters only to me. . . .

Please write soon. . . .

love, Doren

P.S. Andrew sends his love too.

P.P.S. Happy Valentine's Day, Candice, and sentiments of FRIEND-ly love from your truest friend—

love, Doren

———————

My first choice regarding colleges was a small college in Boston where I could major in theater yet receive a liberal arts education. I went up to Boston for my interview and stayed with Andrew and Doren. Doren came with me to the school, walked around with me, coached me on questions I should ask during the interview, and also gave me her advice. She warned me about the rules this particular school had—they were unflinchingly medieval. I didn't listen to Doren's warnings. I had already made up my mind. This was the school I had to go to. Screw the rules. Screw 9 P.M. curfews, notes from a parent to sign out for weekends, freshman hazing, house councils, etc. I would come into this place and immediately begin to politicize. Surely everyone in my dormitory would back me, surely everyone would want the archaic rules abolished. The only certainty was that I was dead wrong. By the time I found that out, I was trapped in that school for one year.

My senior year at Walden ended in a flourish. I was brazen enough to allow the yearbook to publish a couple of my poems and to have a blowout with my competition for Kevin—she had kept me out of the Teachers' Room once too often so I finally threw a fit and began screaming at her in front of everyone. I was just about as cruel as I could possibly be, revealing to her and everyone else that I knew of her feelings for Kevin, her jealousy of me, her marriage which she never acknowledged. The woman trembled before me. I thought she might faint, and I couldn't have been less sympathetic or more coldhearted. When I think now about my behavior, I tremble as she did then. All my anger that had never found an outlet emerged like a trim, purposeful laser beam. I pierced this woman before me whose only sin was that she had, in some fashion, gotten in my way. I was tired of competing, I wanted to grab on to something I did not have to share, or concede, or feel guilty about, or hide.

The summer after I graduated from high school, I worked as a salesgirl at Bonwit Teller's. My first job, my first bank account. I was not excited; I was bored. Had it not been for the discovery of Terry, another salesgirl who was my age, with cynicism equal to mine, I would have quit after the first day. Terry and I entertained each other, ate our lunches on the roof, gossiped during coffee breaks. We kept each other company all summer long, in and out of the store.

I was seeing Christopher, but I was keeping this a secret from my family. I was sure they would disapprove after I had told them we had broken up. Terry tried to talk me into going with her and a group of her friends to the festival at Woodstock, but I wasn't interested. Camping out for days with thousands of people was not something that excited me. Besides, Christopher had suggested I come to Boston during that time and that we hitchhike to Cape Cod to visit friends of his. This idea sounded far more appealing and romantic than a crowded outdoor concert.

I will always regret my decision. Not because I missed out on my generation's historical high point, but because on the way to Cape Cod, having hitched a ride with a woman driving a red VW beetle, I was in a car accident. No one was seriously injured, but it was bad enough and bloody enough to render the experience traumatic. The woman driving had a small cut on her forehead and was dazed. I had whiplash. Christopher, in the passenger seat, hit the windshield and broke his nose. This wasn't apparent at the time. The only thing apparent was the abundance of blood pouring down his face. I thought of every movie and television show I had seen and told myself to stay calm and announce loudly, "Someone call an ambulance!"

Once at the hospital, our parents had to be notified. Just my luck. I had lied to my mother about where I was going that weekend and with whom. Now she would find out not only that I had lied, not only that I was with Christopher, but that I was also in a hospital emergency room. I didn't call my mother right away. I called Doren. Doren assured me she would take care of everything. She told me not to worry. Christopher's parents were driving from Boston to pick us up and Doren told me I should have them take me to her house. She and Andrew would be waiting for me. They would take care of me. I would spend the night with them.

Suddenly my priorities shifted. It was no longer of pressing importance that I be with Christopher. He was more than a little insulted that I was choosing not to stay at his house. But I was seeking comfort. And I knew exactly where I had to go to find it.

The car ride home—I thought of Doren and Andrew's as home—was interminable. I felt unsafe, physically vulnerable, thinking about the accident and what *might* have happened. Christopher wanted my sympathy and I couldn't give him any. I was too busy fearing for my own life.

There were soft lights, herbal tea, and a hot bath waiting for me in the one-bedroom apartment in Cambridge where Doren and Andrew lived. Although the hospital had given me a tranquilizer, I was jittery as hell. I was guilty about leaving Christopher, apprehensive about my mother's reaction to finding out I had lied, but sitting at Doren and Andrew's small round kitchen table, I knew that at least I was safe.

Doren and Andrew did not have sleeping accommodations for guests. I suppose they didn't feel right, considering I had just been in a car accident, to have me sleep on the floor or scrunch up on their Naugahyde love seat. The only other option was to share the double bed with them.

This made for comic relief. Who would believe, we thought, it was all as innocent as it was? Of course we all thought it was perfectly innocent. With Doren in the middle, the three of us lay facing in the same direction. Snuggled into each other in spoon positions was all there was room for. When someone wanted to turn, we all had to turn. When this occurred, Andrew would sing the pronouncement, "Wagon-ho-ohhh."

Although reluctant to leave my safe harbor, I returned to New York the next day. I was surprised to find that my mother did not scold me about lying, she was simply relieved that I was all right. I was happy that within a matter of weeks I would be living in Boston and could see Doren and Andrew as often as I wished.

I never realized how traumatic it would be to leave my mother in the fall of 1969. We clung to each other desperately, frightened of the dangers that might befall us if we were to let go. Having anxiously awaited the moment that would initiate my independence, I was more than a little surprised to find myself hanging on for dear life when the time came to take my leave.

I sobbed. Mother sobbed. She sat in my room watching as I did my last-minute packing. I pleaded with her to stop crying. I couldn't stop if she didn't. She kept apologizing and repeatedly said, "I know I'm not supposed to be doing this." I wondered why we were acting as if we would never see each other again. I tried to make light of the mysterious terror that gripped us both. I said, "Don't think you're rid of me *yet*," and she said, "What will I do without you?" For just a moment I smiled slightly and said, "Plenty."

Mother came over to hug me. If I could have bronzed us in that embrace, I would have.

I left my mother's home and set off for new territory. In that new land, my sister was waiting for me.

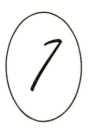

To get to Doren and Andrew's apartment, I have to walk through Harvard Yard. Always, whatever mood I am in changes once I am in Harvard Yard. I become humbled. I feel privileged to be in this place although I'm not sure why. It is as if every time I visit my sister and her husband I go through a rite of passage. When I emerge from Harvard Yard I feel unusually calm, mature, purposeful. When I arrive Andrew is usually not home. He often works at his lab until late into the night. Doren ushers me into the kitchen, where she has cooked something she knows is to my liking. We sit at the table and talk and eat. I tell her how miserable I am. She gives me advice. I am swamped with home-work and I am sure I will never get everything done. Doren offers to do some of it for me. She will draw the designs and costumes for a production book I must do in one of my theater classes. Doren has made it her task to make sure I do not drop out of school and to make sure I do not lose my mind. Later, we lie on her bed watching sitcoms, and we laugh.

The dining room in my mother's apartment is dark even during the day. Doren has cancer and spends her days and nights in this room now, lying on a mattress on the floor because it is more comfortable for her than anything else. She no longer wants the nurses, who have been taking care of her in her own home, and she does not want to be alone. She has left her own home for the last time. The doctor has told us Doren is dying. He agrees not to tell Doren outright, but says that if she asks, he will tell her the truth. She never asks. I sit on the floor next to Doren, massaging her hands and feet. She tells me this feels wonderful. It helps to lessen her pain. She knows I have been hav-ing arguments with my father. "Okay, Cathy," she begins, "I'm going to teach you how to handle difficult situations with our father. There are just a few things you need to know." I tell her it's okay, not to worry, everything will clear itself up. "No," she says. "I've always been a lot better at handling things with him than you are. But . . . now it's your turn." I don't hear what follows because what I am thinking is—she doesn't have to ask because she knows. I know she knows.

*E*ntering my freshman year, I was labeled immediately as a troublemaker. With one exception, no one in my dormitory felt the way I did about changing the rules. They were perfectly content to leave well enough alone. The exception was one of my two roommates—the one who, once a week, tried to commit suicide. Her name was Lorena. She was my only friend.

Christopher was attending another college in Boston. He and I were not getting along. We clashed from the moment I arrived. There didn't seem to be anything that could keep me afloat except my buoys, Doren and Andrew. Doren advised me not to take any of the required courses. I was too unhappy to be able to cope with the boredom they would instill. Doren practically demanded I take only courses that interested me. The required credits I could fulfill at a later date when I was more oriented, stable, equipped. I spent my time taking theater classes, literature classes, and choreography classes. All of that was fine. In fact, my freshman year I made the dean's list. This was a mystery to me. Doren helped me so much I sometimes think it was she who made the dean's list. That first year away from home I was exceedingly depressed and panic-stricken.

Doren gave me a key to her apartment so that I could come and go as I pleased. She understood that every minute I spent in the dorm was torture. She had experienced a similar plight at Bryn Mawr. Andrew had no say in my comings and goings. Doren had made a decision: I came first. She actually told me she wanted to make up for the rotten way she had treated me when we were younger. I never really understood what she meant by this. Andrew had no choice but to acquiesce. Doren's determination was not anything he dared to mess around with. Nor could he alter the dynamic between sisters that seems to produce a life of its own.

There was one particular night I realized I was in a great deal of trouble with myself. Lorena and I were lying in our dark room on our beds. Our third roommate, whom we both despised and who despised us, was not there. Lorena was explaining to me, in rational tones, why suicide for her was a viable option. She explained the details of her life that had brought her to this point. Whatever it was she told me made sense. I couldn't think of a convincing argument for continuing on that would top her argument for ending it all. I had been reprimanding Lorena for weeks, not to mention breaking into locked bathroom doors to save her from herself. As it was, her body was covered with bruises. We took a choreography class together, and when learning new combinations, Lorena would fling her body all over the place, not taking care to protect herself until the steps became second nature. She would fall down five times in five minutes. She had even been walking around for weeks with a broken ankle she was neglecting to get mended.

It was shortly after this evening that I heard strange sounds in the hallway after the nine o'clock curfew. I crept out of my room to see what it was. Lorena was sitting on the steps, crying softly. This was no small matter. Lorena's mother had died when she was a young girl, and because she had never cried at that time she vowed to herself that she would never cry for the rest of her life. "If I couldn't cry for my mother," she would tell me, "I certainly have no right to cry about anything else." So Lorena weeping on the steps was a powerful event. She hadn't shed a tear in at least a decade. I sat down next to her, put my arms around her, and began to cry as well.

From downstairs a voice boomed, "Lorena and Cathy, you're dormed!" This was a punishment. It meant we were grounded for however long the House Council (consisting of other girls in the dorm, the House "Mother," and the House Mother's assistant, a very severe senior who belonged to the voice that had just yelled at us) determined. "What for?" I yelled back. "For crying in the hallway after hours." At this the volume of sobbing from Lorena and me increased, and the voice downstairs boomed again. "Lorena and Cathy, you're double-dormed!" "What for?" "For crying in the hallway and disturbing the sleep of one of your dorm-mates!" I had never even heard of "double-dormed." It had just been invented for our benefit.

There was to be a trial. Our country was involved in a war, protests were being organized in Boston, excessive drug-taking among students was an unmanageable problem, and I was being put on trial for crying and waking someone up. I didn't have an attorney to call, but I did have Doren.

Doren convinced our mother she had to fly to Boston immediately to save me from the witches' coven. My mother arrived in a flourish, marched, with me in tow, into the office of the college president, wagged her finger at him, gritted her teeth, slitted her eyes, and threatened him with all she had. Part of her ammunition was to inform him that a reporter for *Life* magazine was ready and waiting to make this a cover story. Did he want the school's name blackened? My mother's tale was a true one. The reporter was a woman she knew. Our demands were that I not serve the sentence put forth by the House Council (staying in my room for an entire weekend—Lorena had been let off, they knew of her suicide attempts and felt sorry for her) and that I be allowed to live off campus. The president reluctantly agreed, but only if I observed the living-off-campus policy—I had to live with family. We informed him I was going to live with my sister and her husband. This wasn't the truth. Or was it?

I answered an ad in the paper and at the beginning of second semester moved into an apartment in Cambridge with two other women. One held séances frequently and had a bolt lock on her bedroom door which she used before leaving the house. The other one forbade me to allow Christopher into the building because his hair was too long. She was afraid he'd scare some of our elderly neighbors. Out of the frying pan and into the fire I leapt. I begged Christopher not to break up with me and I used my key to Doren and Andrew's apartment as often as I felt I could get away with it. I was getting away with it a lot.

Doren worked at Filene's department store as a copywriter. She was so efficient at her job that she usually had many hours free in which to do her own work. Or, for that matter, mine. Doren was starting a novel and her office at Filene's seemed to be the most private place for her to write. I met her for lunch often and we ate in the store's cafeteria. After lunch I'd sit with Doren in her office for a while as I did my homework or she helped me with it. The production book Doren was doing for me was hidden behind her desk. She was doing large elaborate drawings of costumes and sets and, as she told me, having fun with it. I was overwhelmed at how much of her time and energy were being spent on me, and told her, more than once, how grateful I was.

Although Doren's job afforded her time to write, she was not all that pleased with it. She also had a sense that Andrew was being competitive with her writing. She felt he much preferred it when her attentions were being directed toward him.

My job is strange. I find it almost incredible that so many people think of advertising as a vital profession. I must daily conquer my guilt about doing such extraneous work. I ease my conscience by telling myself I will be there only as long as it takes to get into writing full-time. But that is an excuse that always falls short of satisfying. A small compensation—I am getting very good at this job—copywriting—and it is a boost to anyone's ego to know that he/she can do a job—any job—well. The value judgment must be made, however. Is the job *worth* doing well? The answer is certainly no. I've almost decided to aim for a jobless future, strictly speaking. I think the only real satisfaction I will ever have is in creating my own fictions. Which reminds me—I have thought more than once of writing a purely fantastical story for the "novel" —the story of what I would have been if I had decided NOT to get married. . . .

The center of the novel has got to be *intensity* of feeling. Which is why I'm finding it difficult to get under way. I don't feel intense. . . .

————————

It was while I went about the motions of everyday life in a considerable haze of confusion and depression that my old friend Emily convinced me to come to a consciousness-raising women's meeting. Emily was now at Boston University. She was an actress and also a "heavy" in the Women's Movement. Emily had been my only consistent friend in my class at Walden. We were peers, but she quickly became my mentor in two major areas—sex and politics. Emily considered herself a Marxist, and had been, she said, even *in utero*. Her mother, perhaps a member of the Communist Party, had been questioned at the McCarthy hearings while she was pregnant with Emily. This questioning immediately followed the Rosenberg executions. Had it not been the Rosenbergs, Emily told me, her own parents could have been McCarthy's scapegoats.

It took weeks of Emily's coaxing until I finally relented and went to her Tuesday night "collective" meeting. I couldn't help but notice that all the women in the room had hairy legs. Did being a part of the Women's Movement mean you had to stop shaving? And would I have to throw away my mascara?

The meeting was held in a dorm room at Boston University. It was starkly illumined by a fluorescent light and the odor in the room was a combination of soggy sneakers and lemony Jean Naté cologne. The cologne, I was informed later, belonged to one of the women who lived in the room who was still rooted in her oppression. She, of course, was not present at this meeting. There were five or six of us there, and the conversation consisted mainly of complaints about boyfriends and advice doled out. I didn't say a word about myself, but I did offer advice. Another order of business was to plan how to organize the women in the dorm. Leaflets concerning a Women's Rally had to be passed out, and a women's caucus had to be formed for a demonstration at the Internal Revenue Service headquarters. The women in the room who were in the know were fed up with the men in the Vietnam Peace Parade Committee. This Tuesday Night Collective would join forces with other collectives in the area.

Caucus. Rally. Committee. Demonstration. Vietnam. All these words were foreign to me. The women spoke of a drama taking place outside what had always been my own all-encompassing internal drama. One woman was saying something like ". . . that woman on the third floor I told you about who was reading *Cosmopolitan* while I was talking to her about male supremacy. . . . I think we should steer away from terms like 'male supremacy' and 'imperialism' with some of these women. It's a big leap from nail polish to revolution. . . ."

I didn't feel I completely fit in here, but I certainly felt safer with these women than I did in my new apartment with my severe roommates. I began spending nights on the floor of Emily's room. We'd split her bed in half; she'd sleep on the box spring, I'd sleep on the mattress. I took part in meetings, I helped with leaflets, I went to marches. The intensity of my own problems lessened as my anger began to be directed outward at larger injustices like the Vietnam War, and then Kent State.

Doren, in the meantime, was lengthening the hems of her skirts, buying clothes of muted colors, cooking dinner every night for herself and her husband, using the monogrammed towels that someone had given them for their wedding, and entertaining Andrew's colleagues. She was doing everything she felt a wife was supposed to do, and looking the way she thought a wife was supposed to look. Her behavior during that period did not become clear to her until years later. I hadn't noticed her lackluster phase either. It never occurred to me that her marriage could be anything but whole. I still needed it to be perfect. Why did I assume that every woman except my sister was oppressed?

Christopher, who had always been on the side of pacifism, arrived one day looking for me in Emily's dorm. He was wearing a football helmet and carrying a baseball bat. There were riots in Harvard Square and Christopher thought it was about time he joined the aggressive antiestablishment throngs. I was horrified. I was sure Christopher would go down there and get himself killed. I appealed to Emily, who, I felt, was a lot more articulate and persuasive than I. Emily seemed somewhat amused by Christopher. She did not really take him seriously, and she told him simply that he was being ridiculous and it just wouldn't be safe in Harvard Square. "So who said revolution was safe?" Christopher asked, sweat seeping down his face from under the football helmet. Now that I was an expert, having read the *Communist Manifesto* cover to cover, I imparted my wisdom at this crucial juncture—"How do you figure this juvenile behavior in Harvard Square is revolution? For someone who makes such a point of being a member of the working class, you don't seem to have any perspective on the real roots of social change."

Sounded good to me. It didn't sound anything *like* me, but I liked that. I felt I was always the recipient of someone's teaching—Doren's, Emily's, Christopher's—and I didn't know what it was *I* had to offer.

Doren and Andrew began having fights in my presence. Doren, I noticed, was growing increasingly irritable and overweight. I began to feel I was becoming a nuisance to Emily and spent more nights in my Cambridge apartment, peeking out my bedroom door every time I wanted to go to the kitchen or the bathroom, checking to make sure I would not run into either of my roommates in the hallway. I visited my mother one or two weekends every month. I never visited my father. I wanted minimal contact with him and did not understand why. I read my high school journals frequently, and, when I was in the New York apartment, spent weekends going through cartons of childhood memorabilia. I wanted out of the college I was in and felt victimized by. I applied to Boston University for sophomore year and was accepted. The plan was this: I was to live on the top floor of a small, run-down apartment building in Allston with seven other women who were also in the Women's Movement. Emily would be one of my roommates and was the person who persuaded me to join the group. By the time freshman year was out, so too were Christopher and I. The only consolation was that I no longer had a minimum of one sister; my sister quotient had expanded to seven, at the least, and, at the most, to every other female I could think of.

Doren kept herself apart and silent from my rantings and ravings during my "militant" days. I suspect she felt it was a phase I would outgrow in much the same way my mother had felt confident, years before, that one day I would cut the bangs that grew down over my eyes. Neither were completely incorrect.

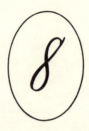

8

It is the summer after I have completed my sophomore
year at Boston University. I am home in New York,
living with my mother and working in her office. I am
now, I know, permanently without Christopher and I
am training myself not to look back. A four A.M. phone
call shatters my summer daze. Doren is coming to stay
with us. Alone. When she arrives her face is blotched
from crying, her shoulders hunch forward in tension.
When she makes eye contact with my mother or me,
she starts to cry. My mother hugs Doren, I hug Doren,
we all hug each other. I feel helpless. How can I comfort my sister? She says she can never go back to Andrew. I can't help but think about Andrew and how
alone he must feel. I tell Doren this. I tell her that
Andrew must be crying too.

I am sitting on my mother's bed, alone in her room
with the door closed. Doren's small, black phone book
is in my hand, the phone is next to me. Doren died
last night. Now I have assigned myself the task of
calling her friends to let them know, and to tell them
about the service we are having for Doren in a few
days. Over and over again I am apologizing—"I'm
sorry to have to tell you this, but . . ." Over and over
again I hear people on the other end of the phone
apologizing—"I'm so sorry . . ." Doren is dead and
we are all apologizing. The person I want to call most
of all is Andrew. They have been divorced for at least
five years. The last time he spoke to Doren was five
o'clock one morning when she called him and blamed
him for the fact that she had cancer. She felt birth-
control pills had caused the disease, and Andrew, she
said, had not wanted her to go off the Pill when they
were married. Accusations didn't matter now. Where
Doren had focused blame didn't matter. I knew
Andrew had loved her. I knew Doren had loved
Andrew. I was the only one in my family who

believed this. Doren had managed to convince everyone it was never true. But I knew better. I had been
around them too much not to know. Andrew will
want to come to New York for the service. I am certain of it. And I am right. My mother is shocked. He
walks over to her at the house afterward and says,
"Doren and I really did love each other. We were
young; we had an intense relationship." Andrew
has remarried, and he shows me photographs of
his two children. I tell him how happy I am he came.
I know Doren loved you, I say. He nods. When
he leaves I know we will never see each other again.
I know he has to leave the part of his life that is
Doren behind.

I returned to New York for the summer following
my freshman year. Before leaving Boston, Emily and I cried
together, helplessly, after returning from a memorial
rally to honor the murdered Kent State students. A mass
strike had been called at Boston University. We felt so small,
so inadequate. I didn't feel I was receiving solace from my
family. Leaving Doren and Andrew for the summer did not
feel difficult. I was angry at them for not expressing their
feelings about the Vietnam War in the same exact manner I
was.

What I discovered during my sophomore year was the
existence of slumlords and the fact that every woman was
not my "sister." It was also during that year my parents'
divorce came through. Doren remained the go-between for
my father and me. Usually I would call on her for assistance
when I needed money. I would be afraid to telephone my
father, aware of how much he resented financing me when
I was refusing to be emotionally involved with him. We
were, of course, emotionally involved, but I was oblivious
to it.

As far as I knew, I had no feelings for, and was in no need
of, a father. Doren was my father's daughter, I thought. I was
not. And, I thought, that was fine with me. The most telling
letter it seemed I ever wrote my father was one when I was
very young. I found it balled up in a carton with Beatles
souvenirs. Written in pencil, in a child's slanted scrawl, everything is printed except for the signature, which is in sloppy
script:

Dear Father

The first thing I want to say is happy birthday. I still Love you even though I never kiss you when you come home from work,

from your
daughter
Cathy Arden

In the apartment house where I lived with seven women, there were three flights of wood stairs that held no promise of taking you where you wanted to go. It required serious navigation to get to the top floor where we lived. Few steps were free of rot and decay and one's foot had to be protected from disappearing into the abyss.

The apartment itself was, at best, ugly. At worst, life-threatening. The ceiling in the hallway fell during a snowstorm and was never repaired. I had all manner of roommates—one woman woke up one day and announced her decision to be a lesbian, whereupon that night she brought home her new girl-friend, who wore a leather jacket and rode a motorcycle; another had a different man sleeping with her every night; another had a boyfriend who was a poet and would bring home street people who needed shelter and drink; another woman felt Emily was being selfish for not sharing her boy-friend with her; another wore abbreviated T-shirts and nothing else, even when there were guests in the house; another cried most of the time; another kept completely to herself and her schoolwork.

I had a lot of company, but I felt terribly alone. Of course I associated none of my sadness with the finalization of my parents' divorce. As, years before at fifteen, I couldn't imagine that my complete disinterest in school and failing grades had anything to do with my parents' separation.

I returned to my mother's home in New York for the summer. My mother gave me a job working in her office. She was now the publicity director of a publishing company. I don't know which brought more comfort—the diversion of a job or the comfort of being around my mother day and night.

It was during that summer Doren's marriage went into crisis. Andrew hadn't returned home one night, and when Doren began calling all their friends' houses, she located him, near dawn, at one particular woman's home. Andrew did not deny he had slept with her.

Doren was in shock. So was I. How could this happen to the

perfect couple? Between my mother and Doren, I heard talk of Andrew's betrayal. Doren had no idea how she was going to get through this, or if she wanted to work it out with Andrew. She left Cambridge immediately and came to New York to be with my mother and me. We encouraged Doren not to leave her husband. Although Andrew had never before been disloyal, and promised he would never be again, Doren felt the betrayal to be complete, final, unforgivable.

————

Dear Candice—

The very bad thing is really 2 very bad things:

1) Andrew's future professor at Yale was killed two weeks ago in a sailing accident (or suicide—no one knows). Therefore—no more job and Andrew has to try to find something to do before September. After having turned down several other attractive jobs last spring!

2) This tragedy sent Andrew into a tailspin, culminating in a particularly abhorrent and humiliating (for me) infidelity four days later.

I ran away to the country house my mother rents in East Hampton, and now I am back home again.

Andrew is, of course, penitent, and swears he'll be good forever if I take him back, but it's not the sex part that bothers me—it's the way he left clues so that I could find him WHILE IT WAS HAPPENING. What a shock.

Anyway, I do still love him—love dies hard, you know. And my women's lib education tells me that my retaliation in kind will serve no purpose whatsoever—so—

Give me advice.

Write right away. (I shy away from telephone calls right now.)

P.S. Get Joni Mitchell's new album, "Blue," and Derek & the Dominoes' "Layla" (Eric Clapton).

P.P.S. Do you think Andrew deserves the treat of visiting your family in Virginia?

. . . Andrew knows me only from *his* side, of course. And . . . it's just like Hesse said—the me I've been for Andrew is not the whole story. . . .

————

Doren decided to return to Cambridge, although with little faith. She would honor her commitment to Andrew and their marriage, although in view of the circumstances she felt that commitment had paled. I had grave doubts she would ever be able to withstand or forgive Andrew's adultery, mainly because I felt my own powers of forgiveness would perhaps be nil under the same circumstances. I wanted them to work things out as much for my sake as for their own. It was more than needing my myth of the perfect and loving couple to survive. I saw marriage for Doren as some kind of safe port. Ever since I had become aware of my sister's darkness when we were children, listening to her smash apples against the bedroom wall, I feared for her well-being. And if she was unprotected, then subsequently I was as well, since my sister was my shield. In addition, if Doren was content in a marriage, the competition I felt with her was held at a safe distance. With Doren neatly tucked away in a marriage, I was free to explore without the specter of my rival's shadow.

9

Doren and Andrew's new apartment in Cambridge is filled with sun. In their living room there are huge sliding glass windows. Trees outside brush against the glass. Doren has been painting the walls all day. She is exhausted, but radiant. We sit in the middle of the living room floor. The room is empty, but it seems full. The trees glisten colors through the glass. "Tell me how much you like it," Doren says. And I do. Later, Doren reads my writing and says I am progressing by leaps and bounds. Andrew reads in silence, then looks up at me and smiles. Finally I am able to share something with them other than anguish. We are all relieved.

When they have to go out, I stay. Mopping the floors while they are gone, I am satisfied when I begin to feel some blisters forming. I know Doren will be pleased. Am I repaying them for all they've done for me by mopping their floors? Their house looks more and more beautiful. I am relieved they are at peace right now with their lives. Doren and Andrew.

It is September 1979 and slightly chilly. The first thing Doren wants to do, after finding out she will be losing her hair quickly once the brain radiation and chemotherapy regimen begin, is to take pictures. She wants photographs taken of her while she still has all her hair. The entire family, which on this day includes an aunt and uncle from Delaware who have driven in to visit Doren, is out on West 10th Street. It is too shady in front of Doren's building, so we walk until we find sunlight. Doren and I pose for some shots together. We are leaning against a signpost. She is looking down at me affectionately. I am looking up at her, in love and in awe. It is like so many of the pictures of us when we were young. The choreography has not changed. What is also the same is that I appear to be frail, she is more robust, healthier. Within a week, I am visiting Doren in her apartment and looking at the pictures, having difficulty imagining that Doren is the one who is ill and I am the one who is well. Silently, she comes into the bedroom and holds out her hand so that I can see what is inside. She is holding a wad of hair. Then she shows me the wastebasket. The bottom is covered with her dark, wavy hair. "It will grow back," I say. She nods. Then she reaches into a drawer and pulls out some beautiful barrettes I have always admired. "Here," she says, "this is a loan."

*T*he plan for my junior year at Boston University was not to live with the group of women anymore. After that experience I could no longer feel that being a feminist required a belief that every woman was my sister and that I should subsequently love every woman because of her gender. As far as I was concerned, I had only one sister and she was enough for me to cope with. I chose to live with someone I had known vaguely from high school. It was a last-minute arrangement. I hoped that my living situation would be less stressful than the year before. My roommate, Anne, appeared incredibly easy-going. Nothing I did in the apartment seemed to bother her. She was kind to me, was amenable to my typing late into the night or playing music at any hour.

Doren and Andrew were together and it seemed I forgot very quickly about what had occurred between them. Doren never talked to me about it after that summer. I just assumed everything was all right now and that she had recovered from the pain of Andrew's adultery. As far as I could see, they were still a couple; they were still there for each other and they were still there for me. Andrew, having left academia, was a chemist at a commercial firm and Doren was working at a nine-to-five job for a woman who held a political office in Boston. She seemed enthusiastic about her job and hoped she would get back to her own writing.

As I was choosing what classes I should take first semester, I decided to pad my schedule with what was referred to as a "gut" course. This meant a course that required little time, minimal effort. There were a few poetry-writing workshops being offered. In order to be considered for one it was necessary to submit a manuscript of ten poems to the professor. I gathered together some poems I had written in high school and deposited the manuscripts at the English Department. I returned daily, waiting for the accepted names to be posted. Getting into one of these workshops was suddenly very important to me. It seemed I had more of an investment than merely wanting a course in which I wouldn't have to do very much work.

One afternoon the lists finally appeared. I searched frantically for my name. The odds were not in my favor. Hundreds of students tried to get into these few writing workshops and only ten per class were accepted. I saw my name and gasped. My first thought was—this must be a mistake.

The weekend before the workshop began, I spent time with friends on their farm in upstate New York. I arrived back in Boston only a half hour before class with no time to go back to my apartment beforehand. I rushed in at least a half hour late, wearing mud-crusted blue jeans, a dirty sweatshirt, and a knapsack on my back overflowing with beets, carrots, and other vegetables I had picked on the farm. Of course, all the vegetables began cascading out of my knapsack as I stumbled into the room. There was a moment of silence as everyone around the long table stared at me. And then the teacher, Mary Carter, continued.

I was right. There had been a mistake. After I had frantically gathered up my vegetables and then composed myself, I heard Mary Carter talking about "fiction fragments" (a.k.a. short stories) to be handed in every week, along with journals to be kept every day, one-page-single-spaced. What was I doing in this classroom? This was a fiction-writing course. I had submitted poetry. Not only was it a class for fiction writers, it was for advanced fiction writers. Not, as I had intended, a gut course. I felt embarrassed. My name had been put on the list by accident. I hadn't been accepted into a writing workshop after all.

I sat quietly, and quietly sweating, until the class was over. Then I went up to Mary Carter. "Excuse me, but I'm afraid there's been a mistake." She looked at me but didn't say anything. "My name is Cathy Arden and I was on the list of those chosen for your class, but I submitted poetry. I thought this was a poetry workshop. I'm not a fiction writer." There was panic in my voice. She was still just looking at me. She wasn't even nodding. Then she said, "What is your name again?" I told her. "Oh yes," she said slowly. "Now I remember. It's not a mistake. I read your work and I sensed a strength there." My stomach churned. "I just have a feeling," she continued. I started in with the But's. She interrupted me. "Why don't you just give this a try? Give it a couple of weeks. See what you come up with." I didn't want to do this at all. I was terrified. I didn't argue, though, I just made a quick exit. Before I went out I whispered in fearful resignation, "Okay."

I have always referred to this as the time I came out of the closet as a writer. I went home and started writing feverishly. I was calling Doren in hysterical excitement, reading her my stories over the phone, shrieking over and over again, "Do you *believe* I'm doing this? I can't *believe* I'm actually doing this!"

Doren was one hundred percent supportive. She seemed as excited as I was. She became my editor, pointing out first what was wonderful and then offering constructive criticism. She was always gentle. I agreed with her on most of her corrections. When I gave her something to read she would write in soft pencil in the margins. This was in contrast to Mary Carter's red pen slashings and comments across the page—I kept hoping my writing would please her and I always felt I came up short. The journal pages had to be handed in, but it was our choice whether or not we wanted Mary to read them. I gave her permission to read mine. One day I snuck a passage in about her, omitting her name—"Do I dare reveal my impressions of her in the pages of this journal? She seems so incredibly strong, yet so vulnerable. . . . Her laugh gives her away. I deal with her cautiously. . . . I remain in the shadows, observing."

As I was seeking approval from my writing teacher—an external sign telling me it was okay that now I was writing out in the open, risking competition with my sister—I was not receiving that sign from my mother. I was still resisting calling my father. Mother was now living with George, the man she had been involved with for many years. Doren and I were never quite sure if they would, finally, decide to live together. Knowing Mother was happy, we were pleased when they did. However, we felt alternately warm and antagonistic toward George. But his approval mattered a lot to us in many areas. One of those was creativity. George is a writer.

Doren and Andrew come over for dinner and we all indulge in my luxurious vegetable farm-food. Doren and Andrew are ecstatic and exclaim throughout the meal. Mother calls as we are finishing. Why is she being so unenthusiastic these days, these days that are so important to me? Doren tells me George said, "Why does Cathy feel she has to write too?" Damn it. Is this his intellectual analysis? Should I not write because other members of my family do? He doesn't have to worry. I'll always maintain my individuality. After all, I've been writing since I was six years old. Now I'm feeling incredibly good, incredibly happy. He does not understand or accept this. Why am I being criticized for something positive? I feel he is influencing my mother's opinion and therefore she cannot enjoy my happiness. I am sad and disappointed. After every phone call during the past two years I've been at B.U. she has asked, "When are you going to tell me something good and not call me in tears?" Well, I finally am and she is missing it.

Doren compensated for what I felt I wasn't getting elsewhere. Even though by writing I was placing myself in competition with her, I never actually expected she would not be supportive. Doren was thrilled that I was finally "doing" school. She had given up on me academically during my high school years and was angry that, as far as she could see, my brain was not in use. My writing course was acting as a stimulus for my other courses as well, and Doren was encouraging me all the way.

I was new, however, to this world of academia and intellectual excitement, and so the joy I felt in writing and studying was tripped up consistently with self-doubt.

> I will always be frightened of school. If I do well, I consider it an accident. Where did these insecurities come from?

> Beginning to have a fear of fiction fragments. I have become stifled by the various criticisms. I keep trying new styles, and working on the faults—until now everything seems to have gone dry. . . . I have a fear of the semester's end. A fear that I will stop writing. Trying to think up ways to take a writing course next semester. I would have to take five courses instead of four. Where there's a will . . .

> Discouraged with my writing. Feeling totally lost. I keep getting disappointed and confused. Doren gives me some honest encouragement, but it isn't she who is confusing me. . . .

> An "A" on my English midterm and I am ecstatic. My professor writes, "This is the best piece of work I remember having read of yours—the knowledge and under-

standing are both deep and subtle." I am in a state of shock. In a state of shock, and giggling. I reread the exam, trying to figure out what I did right. I can't believe this is me.

Doren was still not writing during this time, not even the journal. She was exhausted by her job, and in the evenings she seemed to be growing more and more irritable. She was also gaining weight and would frequently ask me if I thought she looked overweight. She did, but I didn't want to make her feel worse by telling her this. At the time, she was taking birth-control pills. I didn't understand why she just didn't stop taking them.

> Had dinner with Doren and Andrew tonight. Doren seems calmer. Andrew does not go back to the lab. Probably wanted to take advantage of Doren's good mood. We watch depressing shows on television. Doren starts getting nervous. I try on the sweaters she has given me. . . .

There was rarely a time I left Doren's home without a bag of clothes. She was frequently cleaning out her closet and drawers, and always gave me what she no longer wanted. This practice never stopped. I only became choosier in later years.

Another practice that began while Doren and I were in Boston, and would continue for many years, was our taking a dance class together. The first time we did this, at the Cambridge Center for Adult Education, was at Doren's suggestion. She had started a class she raved about and insisted I had to take it too, that it would be a boost for my spirit. It was. The instructor, Reeva, was wonderful, the classes were invigorating. I always looked forward to them. The time spent with Doren before, during, and after the classes was certainly a part of what felt good.

> I ride my bicycle to Cambridge in less than fifteen minutes. And then I have to tune myself into the dance class —mind and body. It is a relief and a release. . . . Doren shows me the article in *The Phoenix* about Anaïs Nin, and a photograph of her taken at the lecture she gave in Cambridge. Doren smiles ecstatically. . . .

> About to leave for Cambridge. Soon to be dancing again . . . These dance classes are really fine. After an

hour and a half, I feel like I am just beginning. More, more. I want excess. "I cannot install myself anywhere yet; I must climb dizzier heights. . . ." (Anaïs Nin).

I am late for my dance class. I love to watch Reeva's body. Everything flows. How nice if when my thoughts and feelings flow, my body will flow too. . . .

The most relaxed I ever saw Doren during that year was in our dance class. I knew her relationship with Andrew was strained, but I did not concentrate on this. For the first time, my energy was going into schoolwork and I was coming up with "A's." Even though Doren was not enthused about herself and her own life, she never slacked in her role of my number one support. She never stopped telling me how proud she was of me. I didn't actually feel like I was competing with Doren—I felt like I was catching up. But while I was just coming into productivity for the first time, Doren was in a slowdown. It bothered her that she was not writing. When she talked about her relationship with Andrew, she would mainly discuss in-law trouble. Given Doren's descriptions, Andrew's parents thoroughly disapproved of her. They did not understand Doren, it seemed, and were highly critical of her. Why couldn't she be satisfied just to be a suburban housewife? Doren stopped having anything to do with them. If Andrew wanted to see them, he'd have to do it sans wife. This was a constant bone of contention between them. Doren felt Andrew was giving in to his parents, and therefore was being disloyal to her. This, for Doren, was the nucleus of the problem: disloyalty.

Before the Christmas break, I spent hours working in the library. My writing class would soon be over.

Just finished my last fiction fragment. I don't want all this to come to an end. . . . I can't let it end. I've gone through two packages of typewriting paper—more than I have used in my entire school career. I am amazed at what I am capable of producing. . . . Again, amazed at finding out that something I have done is good. I am told that the rough draft of my last writing project does not need much work. . . . Professor K. wants a copy of my last paper— Whitman vs. the Romantic Poets. "It's really good," he says, "I want a copy." Why am I so surprised when I achieve? . . . Went to see *The Last Picture Show* with Doren and Andrew. Then feasted at their mini-dream house.

They're still fighting over Andrew's parents. I try to cheer them up, get them off the same old track. . .

The end of 1971: I was up, Doren was down. I was writing. Doren was in mourning for her muse. She edited my work, she cooked me dinners. I hoped that what was good for me now would help to make her feel better about herself. After all, Doren felt that if she had not helped me through the first couple of years of college, I would have dropped out. She might have been right. Her attentiveness was paying off—I was becoming someone she could respect. Now that her major work with me was done, she would have to turn to herself.

But when I think of Doren during that year, I don't think of her sweating over a stove, yelling at Andrew, reading my stories. I see her wearing black tights and a sleeveless black leotard with a zipper up the front, and she is leaping across a wooden studio dance floor, grinning madly; courageous and shining.

And through that year when Doren felt that her creativity was shut away in some dark place she couldn't get to, still, we danced together. When it came to doing combinations across the studio floor, one woman after another, my sister was more daring than I. I would slink into line behind my sister and watch as Doren leapt across the mirrored room, her image multiplied, her body confident, triumphant.

1972. Up until three A.M. last night, searching for a mosquito. My death flashes have been coming frequently. I gasp, and scream, and curse, and jump out of bed, but still have trouble shaking it. There's a call-in show on the radio—"The Right to Die with Dignity." I leave it on. Morbid curiosity? The woman who has called the program has a thick Boston accent. She is Catholic and she has "lost" her eight-year-old son. "Isn't a child lonely up there in heaven without his mother?" There are no priests she likes. She doesn't know if she believes in the Church. Her fear makes me shiver. I sit on my bed, newspaper in hand (the old *Boston After Dark* that already has some bloodstains on it), the bright light on, scanning the walls—searching desperately for that mosquito.

1981. In last night's dream Doren is sitting on the floor, cross-legged. I am sitting at a desk. She is at the foot of the chair. I try to push her away, with my feet, with my hands. She won't budge. And I know, in the dream, that I can't go on with whatever it is I have to do in my life until I get her out of this room. I feel frustrated and angry that she will not move. I can't push her away.

*A*t the onset of 1972, the middle of my junior year at Boston University, I spent my Christmas vacation at home in New York with my mother. I was feeling lonely and bereft and sorry for myself because I did not have a relationship with a man. I was morose for three weeks, until the night before I was to return to Boston. On that night my mother gave a party which she hoped would cheer me up. It did. I met a man with whom she worked; she had been praising him for months. Mother had been wanting me to meet him. One could say she was, directly or indirectly, fixing me up with her friend and colleague. One *could* say, but she never would. A few months

later, during my spring break, Philip and I began a relationship. My mother became enraged. I had crossed a line—I was
her baby daughter and I was entering her world as a grown-
up.

Doren once again was put in the middle between my mother
and me. However earnestly Doren tried to explain to each of
us about the other's feelings, the rift between Mother and me
grew to mammoth proportions. We had never before suffered
this kind of tension; as an adolescent I was too busy clinging
to her to be tempted into a natural rebellion. Now, as I approached my twenty-first year, we were both straining at the
bit. The symbiotic bond was being ripped apart with a vengeance.

I began the arduous task of trying to cope in a relationship
with a man who was ten years my senior, was separated from
his wife, had a young child, and entertained women, other
than me, on frequent occasions. Doren was finally finishing
her novel and wrote in the evenings, preferably while Andrew
was away at his lab. What she really wanted was to have the
freedom to get up at two in the morning and type until dawn.
Andrew, she said, had fierce objections to this. When he slept
he wanted Doren sleeping. Beside him. Content. When the
novel was finished, Doren felt at a loss.

The desolation I feel right now can only be alleviated by the
hope that I may have some talent as a writer and that a) I will soon
lose my "self" once again in writing or b) my "artistic" soul will
hunt down a companion with the necessary ingredients to get me
writing again or c) that I will suddenly see the error of my ways
and become NORMAL—not once more, but for the first time. . . .

I doubt that Andrew really understands the despair I've been
feeling . . . in fact, I doubt I understand it myself. . . .

Most of the time I feel like I'm attempting to recapture something
invaluable which I have carelessly misplaced . . . sometimes I am
convinced I have never been in possession of whatever it is I
assume I have lost. . . .

Lately, I have been scanning the horizon for new prospects, and
this is what I find: 1) The reasonable is unappealing—i.e., worn out,
undynamic. 2) The unreasonable is appealing, but terrifyingly raw.

I have no idea what I might best be doing at this time. . . . Being
married is more or less safe physically, but more or less hazardous
to health—emotionally. And, then, we must admit that the two
are connected, and that even bad sex may be found to be a cause
of cancer.

Sometimes I wonder if I'll ever get out of this. . . . What? Alive. Sane . . .

The pressure now derives largely from the intuited need to equate my destiny with the destiny of another. And a quite alien, quite different human being. This is the thing that fills me with hysteria. Surely it is difficult enough to be a woman and to live from year to year with some degree of integrity without having to throw one's fate in tandem with the fate of a man in another professional and psychic sphere. . . .

At almost twenty-five, I am quite nearly as lost as I was at fifteen. . . . What have I gained in a decade?

A fatuous—two fatuous degrees.

The end of virginity.

The act of love. At least once. Perhaps several times.

One, maybe two friends.

Marriage.

A first novel.

The right to call myself a "professional" writer.

The experience of working, earning a living in various superficial ways.

The experience of knowing a man for five years. Nonstop.

The recognition of the absurdity of academia.

The recognition of my severe limitations.

The experience of watching a friend vanish by suicide. . . .

—————

Doren's friend, Rick, who had recently committed suicide, had been a writer. She had found a way to meet him after reading his first published novel. They seemed to have developed a kinship that was important to both of them. After his death, Doren talked to me about her fear of suicide. Given certain despairing, horrible circumstances, Doren felt she, too, could take her own life. She told me about the time when she was a teenager when this idea seemed to press in on her. I was uncomfortable hearing Doren talk about this. I told her that I was convinced she was being overly dramatic, that she would never make a decision to end her life. But she told me she was not as convinced about this as I was.

—————

The last time I saw Rick we were leaving the MTA island in Harvard Square in opposite directions. I rushed back to him and said, "Promise to keep in touch."

"I promise."

"Good"—he had already turned again and I turned, too, kissing him, just barely, on his right cheek—"because . . . I really love you, you know."

And then I turned first and ran into the Yard.

I ran all the way home and would have cried once inside if Andrew had not been there to scrutinize my white, cold-sweaty face.

Rick returns for a few minutes, to blind me with the light of his eyes, and the brutality of his fate.

Two months before he died, he was trying to reach me—both in Cambridge and New York—and, although he spoke to our mutual friend (as did I), our information on each other's whereabouts never exactly coincided with the "truth." We left messages for each other at various places. We didn't connect.

And then his messages stopped.

And then he aimed one of his father's antique pistols at his own head.

And that's all there is. All there will ever be.

And I am left wondering for the rest of my life: If people like Rick can't make it, why should I even want to try? Survive for who—for what?

What's so good about being a survivor when the most beautiful ones are among the uncounted dead?

During the last half of my junior year, Doren and I were, as the lingo of that era would have it, on separate trips. It seemed I was hooking myself into another life-support system, an unreliable one at that, and that system's name was Philip. Although I still did my work at school, my passion was directed elsewhere. I was taking another writing workshop with another professor, one that bored me, and I found myself coasting, handing in the same pieces I had written the semester before. I had read Doren's novel, thought it was beautiful and brilliant, and so, once again, I felt I could never measure up to her. If any family member asked me whether I intended to return to my acting, I took this to mean they did not support my writing.

I spent frequent weekends in New York, sneaking around with Philip. It wasn't just that I simply thought it best my mother not know I was with him, I seemed to have feared some extraordinary disaster if she found out. It never occurred to me then what that disaster might be. It was, in fact, the mere existence of my mother's anger directed at me. The anger was a result of the separation occurring between us, and it was the separation I was not handling with ease. There were weekends I spent in New York without my mother even knowing. Those were the scariest of all. I imagined countless scenarios of discovery. Perhaps someone she knew would see us, relay the information to her. Perhaps I'd simply see her walking toward me on the street. What would I do? Of course it seemed as if the answer to that was simple. I'd have no choice but to just lie down and die. I didn't want my mother's anger or disapproval. If I had to formulate intricate patterns of deceit to avoid those things, then that was what I would do. And I would have to learn to live with the fear.

I began to wonder whether or not I should continue to inform Doren of my comings and goings. Since we talked almost daily, it would be hard to disguise a few days' absence. For the time being, I had no choice but to trust her. I certainly was not prepared to put any distance between Doren and me. One umbilical cord was already being tampered with. I didn't dare fool with the other.

I wondered how I was going to live with my mother in New York that summer and continue to see Philip. I certainly didn't want to have to return home on those nights, those rare nights, when Philip and I would see each other. The solution was to get an apartment. I found a place in the Village, I found a roommate, I took a part-time job at a publishing company sending out form letters rejecting unsolicited manuscripts, I took some courses at New York University, one of which was called "The Meaning of Death." *That* was the course I got an "A" in.

During those months I wandered around New York with a knapsack on my back. I stayed at my Village apartment approximately twice. It depressed me terribly, though I didn't know why. Perhaps what was depressing me most was the resentment I felt at not being able to live at home. I didn't actually see Philip all that often either, although the relationship continued to consume me. I trudged, gypsy-fashion, from one friend's house to another, depending on the receptiveness of those friends who felt sorry for me.

I have nothing bright to rest my mind on. Everything has taken on a stormy shade. Solace has diminished. Lightning . . . and nothing soothing to view in the glare. Trebor mountains and trees disappeared for me a long time ago. Only Doren sitting on my bed as a comfort. . . .

My mother and George had a house in East Hampton, Long Island, and I spent an occasional weekend there. I was not at all easy at that time in George's presence. We would argue over small things, and I blamed the tension between us on him. I thought he was having trouble accepting me. I never thought it might be the other way around. I was living my life in my head, constructing formulas, trying to make sense out of them, making shifts in my imagination I couldn't make in real life. My retreat from my life took on a life of its own. During that summer, I wrote to Doren.

Doren—

Probably, in writing to you, I won't be as free as if I were writing in my journal. Things will obviously be a bit shaded since you are my sister with your own biases and prejudices concerning me and the rest of our family. But I have to get a lot of things out (or on paper, at least), and I feel more productive communicating to you rather than to myself in a journal, or to a friend on the telephone who doesn't understand my situation in the first place. I fear that what is bothering me goes further, deeper, than anything I am aware of. If that is so, then neither of us have the capabilities, knowledge, or insight to expose it. Or maybe the things I *know* bother me, bother me even more than I realize. I doubt that, though. There is something that has roots in the darkness of my brain. It is completely unknown to me. . . .

Things are very tenuous and haphazard with Philip. I'm afraid to tell you the details. I don't want you to be down on him. That will leave me worse off than I already am. It's bad enough Mother disapproves of him. . . . What bothers me most of all is that I do think very highly of myself, I think I'm pretty terrific, but with Philip I don't feel that way most of the time. I enjoy *him* when I am with him, I enjoy myself being with him, but I don't enjoy *myself*. . . . I want to fill my life up with other things. Perhaps Philip will become less important. But for the past forty-eight hours I have felt paralyzed. . . .

One weekend I went with a friend to her parents' beach house in another part of Long Island. We went out to a coffee house one night and I spotted a young man who mesmerized me. He looked like an "artiste," with the requisite beard, long hair, wan, sculptured face. He reminded me, in fact, of Christopher. Eric and I developed a friendship. He was my first authentic male friend.

I couldn't have known when Eric came to visit me in Boston that fall that he and Doren would get along so well. And that subsequently Doren would develop a fantasy about Eric I would never know anything of until reading about it, after she died, in her journal.

Things that have been plaguing me for the last few days: My longing for children. A baby. Cathy's ambivalences and hostilities toward me. The entrance of the beautiful Eric, who read my book (just a little) and said *nothing* by various strange accidents, and who—when scolded by Cathy for his apparent callousness—not only expressed belated admiration for the work, but also begged for my address so he could properly explain his behavior—or lack of it—to the author. Cathy told him that wouldn't be necessary. (No comment.)

I suppose I decided earlier today that Eric would be a problem for me in one way or another, hopefully just a head problem, and not an "actual" one. Because he seems entranced by my sister, and because I was similarly entranced by him. I won't even go into the why. That's just the way it is. And, unlike the brazen Cathy, I will do everything in my power to control my passions in order to preserve the familial peace and tranquility.

Cathy has finally released my address to the insistent Eric. . . .

I've begged Cathy for the privilege of writing to Eric, who is in the hospital for minor surgery. And now that permission has been granted, I will write—hopefully, in the next hour.

The only competition that had ever been spoken of between Doren and me was mine with her. I never imagined Doren competing with me, and had it come at me full speed ahead like a tornado, I would still have remained oblivious to the phenomenon. Reading about Doren's infatuation with Eric, in her journals, startled me. I began to turn the pages slowly, uneasy about what I might find. How far did the competitiveness go? As I read about Eric I wanted to pick up the phone and dial his number. We had not been in contact for many years. "Eric, I've just been reading Doren's journals. Listen," I imagined saying, "did you and my sister have an affair?"

Who was Doren? At that time she was more my sister in my eyes than a woman in her own right. What was the marriage really about? I thought it was about what I saw week to week during those Boston years. Where was the truth? Do Doren's journals reveal the truth? To what extent does the voice I am hearing in those journals veer off subtly into concealment?

I search for answers. One day, for instance, I find a name and phone number in her appointment book. I don't recognize the name, but next to the name she has written in parentheses "air conditioner." There is a story Doren told me about a man she had briefly come to know while she was ill with cancer and undergoing chemotherapy. She didn't socialize very much and there was a great deal of tension between her and her boyfriend. It was almost summer and her air conditioner needed repair. A friend gave her Carl's name. Doren told me she would never forget Carl. He had done something for her no one else had, including her boyfriend. Doren wore silk scarves on her head to hide her baldness. She would not allow anyone to see her without hair. What I didn't know, until she told me about Carl, was that she never took the scarf off, even in bed. While making love with Carl he asked if she would remove the scarf. She wouldn't. She was too afraid and ashamed. He told her she had no reason to be and, with sensitivity and gentleness, Carl eased the scarf off my sister's head. Then he told her she was beautiful.

Doren would never forget this gesture, and neither would I. What Doren had also said was that he was more my "type" than hers. To some degree she felt bad that she had met him first. "He's really more for you, Cathy, than he is for me. You'd probably like him a lot." I had not forgotten that. She had never told me his name, though, and when I thought of him years after Doren died, I had no idea how to find him. Now I was staring at her appointment book—"Carl (air conditioner)," with a phone number tagged on.

I called Carl. He hadn't even known Doren had a sister. He had heard Doren had died. I didn't know know what to say to him. So that's what I said. I did say he had done something for Doren that meant a lot to her, and so, too, it meant a lot to me. He asked if I wanted to meet. I said yes. My fantasies leapt like flames. Would I like him, would I sleep with him, would I love him, would I spend the rest of my life with him? Was Doren maneuvering all of this? I felt guilty. As if Doren were still alive. As if I were being disloyal. I was imagining something I never could have imagined, knowingly, while Doren was alive —making love to a man she had also made love with. I felt devious, ridiculous, hopeful.

Within twenty minutes in Carl's presence, I began to choke uncontrollably. On nothing. On no solid matter, that is. I couldn't catch my breath. I stumbled over to the bar in the restaurant where we had met, gesturing wildly that I needed water. It seemed forever before my coughing subsided. I was uncomfortable when I began to sense that Carl was attracted to me. The major topic of conversation was, of course, Doren. He told me how shocked he was to learn of her death, that when he knew her she had told him she was doing so well, that she was recovering. "I thought, when I heard the news she had died, that perhaps her family had misled her—that she was not told how ill she really was."

Perhaps what I was really after with Carl had to do with seeking comfort, a way to connect with Doren, yet another attempt at trying to breathe life into her. But anger took over. Carl was angry about Doren's death and was looking for someone to blame for it. His accusatory comment sent me reeling. My own anger took hold. It didn't matter that what he said was untrue—what mattered was I didn't get the comfort, the connection with Doren I was after. I never saw Carl again.

So much for fantasy. So much for trying to find the truth. If I try to find the truth, or try to find Doren, I find I am groping. I become stuck. Doren becomes a non-person, the person I am creating in these pages. Where is Doren separate from me? Where am I separate from Doren? I am in the present, with all my individuality, and then I find myself going under, into the past. The present becomes only a mirror for what has come before.

I can't make Doren be alive. I foolishly try to, feeling that she is not alive now in her own right. I am picking and choosing, piecing together what once was a human being. I don't know what the truth is. And yet I don't want to be wrong. How could I possibly expect to relate the truth about sisters, about these sisters, about that relationship, about the relationship ending, about that relationship never ending, about Doren being alive with me even now, and me being alive with Doren? How can I possibly explain that which is unexplainable?

I feel inadequate. As I did in the past, trying to weigh myself

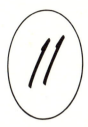

11

It is the year of the gold star. John Barth has accepted me into his writing workshop. I meet Meg. She is in Barth's class as well. We write stories and put gold stars on each other's forehead. Doren reads our stories and puts gold stars on her favorite sentences and paragraphs. Meg and I understand each other. My sister understands us. When I am home for Thanksgiving vacation Mother doesn't understand. Doren and Andrew are there too. I am eager to show Andrew a short story I have just written. I tell him I still have work to do on it, but that I am anxious for feedback. Mother tells me I shouldn't do this. I don't know what she means. She explains, "Doren never shows her work to anyone until it is completely finished. And Doren is the writer." I have a dish towel in one hand, a wet wok in the other. I hurl the wok across the kitchen. "What am *I?!*" I scream, "*—shit?!*" My ears vibrate from the crash of the wok and from the rage pounding in my head. "FUCK YOU!" spills out of me and thrusts me from the room. Doren is not home. Meg is not home in Boston. There is no one to talk to. My story sits on my tiny childhood desk in my old bedroom and I can't find any gold stars.

Doren and Andrew have bought a stereo. Doren is a changed woman. She sits in the middle of the living room floor, wrapped in an afghan, wearing furry slippers, a pair of headphones over her ears, swaying, grinning. I watch her from where I sit on the Naugahyde couch, editing one of my short stories, and I start to laugh. With Joni Mitchell music blaring in her ears, Doren asks me loudly, "Why are you laughing at me?" I don't answer because she wouldn't hear me and anyway I don't have an answer. I just keep laughing.

I was startled to discover that Mary Carter had, after all, admired my work for her class. I received a letter from her at the end of the semester attached to the final project I had submitted—"Your improvement over the semester has been impressive," she begins. I must have stared at that sentence for twenty minutes before continuing. "There's little, really, I can make in editorial comment on your project-piece: you put it together splendidly, developed the logic, expanded the layers, brought us through into the moment of insight. As you know, the technicalities of shaping a whole piece are entirely outside the material of the course . . . here you exhibit a grasp of them entirely on your own. And you've developed an attack and style of your own which is a true one. . . . It was a pleasure to have you in the class. . . . Congratulations on an excellent job."

I don't remember sharing this letter with anyone but Doren. I'm surprised I didn't send it along to those I felt did not accept me as a writer. After the incident with my mother over Thanksgiving vacation, I don't think I talked with her at all about my writing.

At the outset of my senior year I submitted a manuscript of short fiction to a small workshop that was going to be taught by Visiting Professor John Barth. I wanted to get into that class so badly my intense wishing was akin to prayer. Lo and behold, I was accepted.

Doren was envious that I was taking a writing class with Barth. I don't think, however, that either of us acknowledged her envy. I would come back with reports of each class to her. One day Doren popped the question—would it be all right with me if she sat in on one of my classes? I don't recall hesitating when I said, "What a wonderful idea!" I didn't see the danger, at the time, of fudged boundaries. Of course I would want to share this experience with Doren. If I was benefiting from my class with Barth, why shouldn't Doren do the same? She had started writing again and we were both on a similar writing-high.

Doren didn't just come to one class. She came to many. As her journal would indicate, John Barth became a central figure for her that year. I didn't know this, but I began to feel uncomfortable with her presence in the workshop. And I didn't know how to stop something I had helped initiate.

Rushed sweating to rendezvous with John Barth; arrived panting loudly, dripping with sweat and looking far from good. . . . He's casually professorial in beige shetland and gray flannel. . . . Genial, self-effacing, and articulate . . . Stories are read by a guy named Raydon: self-indulgent trash. Or as Barth describes the uncharacterized protagonist: "Despair with a first name."

JB loves Kafka and is referring to the journals in which Kafka displays himself to be a sort of "proto-Robbe-Grillet," with his working and reworking of images and phrases. . . .

"A rage of order"—JB's explanation of his hope that certain of Raydon's lines were in fact song lyrics. "I'm insisting on a unity in your work," Barth confesses with a smile.

"I love the idea of impossibly brief fictions." His gentle lead into a comment that the piece is too fucking short.

I can't keep up with the beauty of his language, of his thoughts. It is so incredible that a man can speak as creatively as he writes. . . . I will have to think more on this.

I love to watch him being himself. Because every human attribute makes him dearer to me. . . . Chewing on a tightly folded, cigarette-sized piece of paper. . . . Gently running his fingers over the curves of his two ball-point pens, side by side on the table. . . . The way his eyes dance when he is amused. . . . The paleness of his skin and hair (that which remains). . . . Truly, I delight in every aspect of his presence.

End of class. Brief dialogue with JB. I tremble with joy. Finally —"I really enjoyed the class." "Thank you." His eyes lower and he scurries (soundlessly, thanks to Hush Puppies) down the hall. . . .

Dear Mr. Barth—

Thank you for letting me visit your class two weeks ago.

After three years of solitary struggle with the art of the novel, a few hours in that particular time and place was something like a stroll through Eden.

Please accept a compliment from this unverified source: I've experienced similarly structured writing courses at Bryn Mawr, Barnard, and Harvard, and not one course, not one session, was ever generated with anything approaching the benevolence and wisdom of yours.

I believe your starting point is something like: that person took time to write it, that person cares about it, therefore, let's help him/her find a way to realize as fully as possible the initial aspiration. Recalling those moments in my ivied past when some teacher or other announced that an opus of mine was "Shit" or even just "Dreadful," I beam with empathetic gratitude on behalf of your lucky students who will not be severed from their possibilities in such a pointless way.

. . . I want to tell you two more things, one which you may know, and one which you certainly do not.

1. You are an exceptional teacher and an exceptional man.

2. *End of the Road* has done incredible things to and for me and my writing.

Best regards—Doren Arden

Cathy first called my careful editing of her story "a hatchet job," then, as she cooled, admitted my criticisms were legitimate and, what's more—that my "good's" and "yeses" were written over the same lines as JB's "good's" and "yeses."

A wonderful thing has happened to me through Cathy today. John Barth told her with real delight that her sister had written him a letter, and then he proceeded to ask her all manner of questions about me, my life, my writing.

Am I married?

Who is representing my manuscript? Are they doing well by it? (C said, in fact, no.)

And C said, too, that when she told him the signs of my writing-high—my going up to people on the street, carrying around scraps of paper to write on at odd moments, etc.—he was laughing out loud with the pleasure of recognition.

Also wonderful is the fact that he told C he has already answered my letter.

The mail yesterday was such a good trip. So wonderful to see the happiness and excitement between the lines of Eric's letter from New York (which included the word "love"—as in "love to see you"). . . .

Barth's letter didn't come, but I can handle that as long as I remember that at the end of the weekend I'll have something to look forward to. . . .

John Barth's note was short, but sufficiently uplifting. He's invited me to sit in on the class "whenever" I "feel like it." One of the finest compliments I have ever received.

Six-thirty A.M. appears to be my new point of departure. It's nice, because I get to see so many sunrises this way.

Cathy told me Sylvia Plath used to get up every morning before the rest of her family and I shouted, "Don't tell me any more! I don't want to count the ways that I resemble Sylvia Plath!"

Which reminds me of another reason why John Barth is center stage in my imagination (fantasies) right now.

He is a real person—a real man. As well as being a writer of genius. He's got a wife and, apparently, four or five pretty solid, nearly grown children.

I want to be able to do what he has done. (Minus the genius, I guess, since I don't expect to have *that* going for me.)

I don't want to be one of the wretched of the earth.

I don't want to be Rimbaud, Plath, Baudelaire, Woolf, Joyce, etc.

I would like to be something like Ms. Nin, M. Barth, even Old Henry Miller—who at 80 looks like 60 because he is HAPPY. FULFILLED. ETC.

I don't want to be the in-terror person I've been for the last 5 years. I don't want to cling to marriage as a lifeline. I want to cling to my talent, whatever it may ultimately amount to.

I WANT TO BE A WRITER.

The prayer rises up from the choked and choking center of my chest and courses through my body, rearranging the molecules of my blood, getting me high and hyper-everything.

———

How could I resist the new choreography? Now Doren was admiring aspects of my life, so much so that she wanted to take part. There was her attraction to my friend, Eric, her admiration of John Barth, her amusement and respect for my new friend and writing buddy, Meg.

> Meg is my friend. We sit, in class, on either side of John Barth. Meg brings me a pumpkin and chicken soup when I am feeling blue. She teaches me how to carve the pumpkin (my first) and buoys my confidence so that I can do it myself. She teaches me how to play the recorder, how to do ski exercises, how to repot my plants. She stays on the phone with me for two and a half hours when I have a lot to say. She comes in her car to see me. We sing songs (I play the guitar, Meg beats a rhythm on my television stand, bed, and dresser), we dance, we talk about deep things, and we type. Meg says, "When I talk to Cathy it's like talking to myself except I get an answer." Meg and I laugh alike. We are amazed we have found each other. It is joyous and festive, and we're celebrating.

Meg is kin. Meg and I are inseparable and it is not unlike the bliss I felt with my sister when we were children. The innocence before the shake-up. Meg and I deciding, at midnight, to drive to the mountains. We are the only car on the dark, wintry road. The song that keeps playing on the radio is "Ventura Highway." We are either silent or, when we look at each other, our grins turn into bursts of laughter. When we return from New Hampshire, we sit in Meg's car in front of her house. I can see her bedroom through the bay windows on the first floor, the walls midnight-blue like the walls in my apartment she had admired so much. I watch the ice melt and drip down the windshield. The motor is off. A few people pass by. Their footsteps are silent. Now we're listening to Bach on WBUR. Meg's eyes are closed and she says she is thinking out a good idea for a story. I am thinking about me doing what I want to do in my life and loving it. Mostly I think about writing.

It is the first time I am living alone, but Meg is often around. She suggests we share an apartment to pool our measly funds, but I want to live alone. There was a relief I felt the first night in my apartment. It is just me now, I remember thinking. My first sense of feeling self-contained, my first glimmer of independence that felt like freedom. As long as I can live alone, Meg's presence is a plus.

Flunked a geography exam today, but who cares! Not me! Because now I am sitting at my new desk, supplied by Meg, in my living room in my apartment. My wonderful apartment. Meg is reading *MS.* magazine on the bed/couch. Fine. This is all so fine. Hung a plexiglass shelf on the window for my plants—shelf also supplied by Meg. Dear friend. Writing at my first real desk. I am grateful for Meg and all she brings. We put together a satellite multicolored mobile. Now there are flowing colors through the room.

I made one comment in John Barth's class last week—to a girl named Meg. I couldn't hold it back. I told her exactly how I thought her piece should—or could—be developed. John Barth thought the suggestion sound, and yet assured Meg that she could also discover a way to handle it in the initial vein. I didn't really agree that that would be a very helpful way for her to go at it. Especially as a young and untrained writer. I felt I could already see in the piece (and in her face) the desperation of the dead end. . . . Anyway, Cathy told me a few days ago that Meg is taking my advice and is really pleased with the results so far. I think she described the flow to Cathy as "magical." . . .

Conclusion of tale: I am elated to rediscover there really are some things I do quite well.

Pleasurable evening with the aspiring Meg. She's delightful and, I have to say it, reminds me quite a bit of me—her energy, her curiosity about life in general and her own limits in particular, her intensity, her inadvertent humor—as when she told the story of her recent mugging a trifle too heavy on the dynamics and hurt her hand on the table.

Meg has practically memorized *Play It As It Lays*. She recited one entire paragraph as she exited.

Cathy and Meg arrived at dinnertime last night with stars in the middle of their foreheads. And the joy in their play made me painfully aware of my nostalgia for the days when Candice and I lived together. In a sense. At Bryn Mawr.

Couldn't finish my own writing last night because friends of Andrew's arrived for dinner, Meg and Cathy called repeatedly for writing advice, and, finally, Doren's fountain of energy trickled into sleep.

Now I will read "Take It on the Rocks," written by Meg. . . . Yes, it is pretty damn good. And my advice was extremely helpful to her. How gratifying that she took it and used it so intelligently.

"Meg really tried to kill herself years ago," Cathy tells me. "It wasn't just a story."

"Yes."

"What do you think about that?"

"Well—I can't be shocked. I've been through it myself. Remember the apple days? I was suicidal then. For example."

Meg has submitted her story to magazines. I will be green if she gets her piece of fiction published before I am published. . . . Cathy's new story re the pain of Philip is called "Fertility Rite."

Very, very good and at the same time it is very, very rough. And even, at times, inept. What she needs is the discipline to struggle with it. To strive for her own level of perfection. But I don't know if that's something she can or is willing to do.

Cathy is experiencing a creative burst, at least partially attributable to a chain reaction set off by Meg and me. I don't think it's bad, though. The competition. As long as it brings fruit. Which brings happiness.

Dear Cathy—
While reading "Periphery" for the second time I found I couldn't resist the reflex to scribble a little minor advice. Hope you don't mind it.

As I said, it's incredibly more careful and aware—in terms of craft—than the last piece and as such deserves three cheers. (Hip Hip Hooray for Cathy!)

One thing of slightly larger importance: I noticed that sometimes the sentence order of paragraphs was (seemed) not quite right and I think it would be good if you read it over carefully just to be sure you are saying things in the *order* you want. Maybe you won't like the order I've imposed in various places—that's O.K., but I'd like to feel sure you've said it *precisely* the way you meant it.

Thank you for sharing another moment of beautiful growth with me.

Love and *respect*,
Doren

I thought Doren's high had only to do with the fact that she was writing again. I was relieved to see her happy, though I recall feeling somewhat concerned about her still, and edgy in her company. I wondered how long the high would last. I didn't know about another new development—Doren had decided to look outside her marriage for male companionship.

The stereo was the turning point. My life now is accurately described as pre- or post-stereo. As Cathy pointed out, the machine didn't effect the change—I did, when I elected to get it. In any case—as I used to say—the stereo started by re-sensitizing, re-eroticizing me, ears first, and many things followed from that. What was lovely was that it felt almost as if I was being acted upon by some mysterious, benevolent force, opened up slowly and delicately like the petals of the imaginary flowers Lillian, the dance teacher Cathy and I had as children, used to ask us to pretend we were at the start of dance class. . . .

And now I've even got a 25-foot extension cord for the headphones. I am so glad to be sitting on the most comfortable furniture in the living room, feet up, journal in lap, cuddled neck to ankles in a heavy winter robe, headphones on tight and Brahms echoing through my cranium. And all without enraging Andrew. Now, if only I can find a way to muffle my electric typewriter so that I could be typing now. (The cord reaches to the desk.)

I made a fabulous French stew for dinner—four hours of cutting, measuring, stirring, tasting, loving—and neither Andrew nor Cathy really dug it the way I wanted it to be dug.

And, though I know it was superb, I cannot be happy just knowing for and within myself.

Dear Candice—

. . . I am alive, I am experimenting (both with and without Andrew's knowledge) and, most important, *I AM WRITING*. Also, I have a very fine semipolitical, good-paying job. . . . And I have made the acquaintance of John Barth, who is *the most fabulous older man* I ever set eyes (and ears) upon. . . . My life is suddenly so intricately beautiful I find it difficult to go through all the stages —to explain step by step how I got where I am now. To allay your fears, however:

1) It does not involve drugs.

2) It does involve sex, but only secondarily, e.g., sex and good music (the new stereo) are about equally significant (but minor) components.

3) The fact of being 25—a kind of delayed reaction over the way I've been sleepwalking through my own life—precipitated the whole metamorphosis. . . .

Which is really what has occurred. I'm 15 lbs. lighter, truly better-looking, more graceful, more everything.

In fact, if this weren't Election Day, I'd be dancing around my apartment to the new Cat Stevens album, one side of which is extremely sensual and danceable. . . .

Write to me, but not too blatantly, because Andrew sometimes peeks at my letters when I'm not looking. . . . Love, Doren

I keep telling people, "You don't know the half of it." Cathy, Andrew, Mother, etc. Probably some people know half, or even a little more than half, but that isn't enough. I really need someone who knows the whole.

No, no, no. I can't fool myself about love. . . . I believe I truly LOVE, for example, my mother, Cathy, and Andrew because I can sometimes put their happiness ahead of my own.

These last two weeks of high have brought me closer to Cathy. Very. And that makes me happy, although we have, naturally and consequently, experienced a great deal of pain because of each other.

Cathy asked if one could be "in love" with two people at once. "Yes or no," she demanded. "Well, yes, as long as you forget about love and call it something else. Anything else."

Andrew and I were watching a television drama the other night and when the police sergeant described the outward manifestations of amphetamine addiction, Andrew looked at me quizzically and we both laughed out loud: hyper-talkative, incessant sweating, unquenchable thirst, dry mouth and lips, inability to sleep, etc. "Andrew," said I, "I'm not popping amphetamines, if that's what you think." "But, Doren," said he, "your body is producing a pretty good amphetamine all its own."

Doren was experiencing, in her own words, "a reawakening." With this came feelings about her own mortality and a resurgence of her need to have children. She was frequently saying, "I don't know where my children are going to come from." I didn't ask why she was not having a child with Andrew. As far as Doren was concerned, the time for that had come and gone. I don't think Doren was looking outside her marriage for sexual adventures. The more pressing adventure for Doren was to find the father for her children.

I walk around the house, through stores, in subways and buses, all the time thinking, Let me carry your baby, and I don't even know who I am talking to.

I am longing for a child—e.g., for ten minutes late yesterday afternoon I watched a young mother and her four-year-old son. When I glimpsed the utter joy and abandon with which she invested a kiss on that boy's cheek, I felt tempted to jump through the glass doors—and all physical and metaphysical impossibilities—right into her maternal shoes. It appears to be unspeakably lovely—moving about the world accompanied by a little piece of one's own flesh, I mean.

Babies. An important thing on my mind. Like—on the bus, I noticed for the first time some retarded children playing with their teachers in a little pocket park near my home.

I almost jumped out of the bus and offered my volunteer services a few afternoons a week. The urge was censured by my laboring "reasonable" faculties—they said why on earth should anyone seriously consider a nut off the street who breathlessly offers her help ("What's she *on*, anyway?").

But I still might follow through because I can see I'm experiencing quite an intense baby episode right now. And I need to preserve myself from reckless acts. . . .

As I said to Cathy (Jesus, it sounds like I've been talking to her nonstop), not only have I suddenly been hit with my age and the fact that if I'm ever going to have biological children it really ought to be in the next five years . . . but also because I've finally admitted to myself that the feeling I need (want) for baby-making has come and gone between me and Andrew. . . .

All I can think is that I really ought to do a trick—like the retarded children-volunteer thing—to satisfy my need for kinder-propinquity. Until I do, I'll be crying over babies in the street, and contemplating the advantages of kidnap.

I remember describing Cathy to a new friend and telling him— "She is prettier by far than me." He looked at me in true disbelief.

"How could ANYONE be more beautiful than you?"

And something electric coursed through my body when he said that—not because I could believe it as objective truth—I didn't— but because I could see that HE believed it. I haven't been the same since he said that to me. . . .

How could I dare let Andrew come near me? It would be cheating; that is, it wouldn't be HIM, and I don't want him to misunderstand. Nor do I want that confusion and guilt. . . . I am angry at him, ever since he betrayed me. I don't want to—and am unable to—afford him access to my body. At this time. He says he is reconciled to this. Even chooses to recall that we made love within four hours of our first meeting and that, in the light of that, it seems fitting to be finally having a courtship. Even if it is 5½ years later. And just about one month before our fourth wedding anniversary.

Cathy called last night especially to say she had just made a barley soup and that it was good and she felt "just like a mother."

I am beginning to see that I may not feel "just like a mother" until I convey a passion-conceived baby through my own "special opening," as Mother used to tell me when she was big with Cathy and I was three.

People are getting to me. . . . The man in the shoe-repair shop who is *always* kind to me—and not in the ugly, chauvinist way. . . . The acute sensitivity of Eric . . . Cathy's vulnerability . . . Andrew's, too, for that matter. . . . Sometimes I wonder if I'm strong enough not to die from intensity. . . .

Cathy dreamt a fearful dream that I was dying and that I walked around saying—"Don't touch me. Don't talk to me. I have to find a way to romanticize this."

I laughed into the telephone because the shock of recognition was too searing to do otherwise.

It was that year, too, that Doren became preoccupied with a dread fear of cancer. Breast cancer specifically. It appears that this fear had its roots in her adolescence.

. . . sitting in the backyard, listening to all the relatives discuss life via minute details such as clothing and children. Is that what it will be? Vague pride of children, exaggerated gaiety to smooth over buried fears? Aunt Jan sits stiffly in a sleeveless suit but her scar shows anyway. It must continue from her left shoulder to the center of her chest, swing around and around where a breast should be. . . . I become frightened and run upstairs to one of the bedrooms. I've locked the door. . . .

My left breast is swollen terribly. It's very frightening. Mother says it's glandular. . . .

I'm going to the gynecologist. . . . He's going to examine my tender left breast and tell me if he'll have to amputate or not. . . . Well, maybe that's an exaggeration, but I'm so afraid I can't even think about it. . . .

One night—in a confessional mood—I told Allyn that I feared breast cancer more than I feared death. He led me into the kitchen, where his mother was washing our dinner dishes. She turned and smiled at us. Then Allyn led me back into the living room and announced that his mother had had a mastectomy and "Look at her—she's all right, isn't she?"

_____

After that early scare as a teenager, the fear stayed with Doren. While she lived in Boston she was continually coming into contact with women who had had breast cancer. Doren feared that if any disease were to get her, this would be it.

_____

Mother has told me that a former high school friend of mine had breast cancer. She is one of the few females I have ever envied in my life. What can it mean? How can I give thanks for being spared thus far? No way. The absurdity of the universe, far from producing nausea, sends a semisexual shiver of fear down the back of my neck.

Another aunt has had a breast removed. I didn't even realize she was "my family" until Cathy shrieked in pain and said, "Oh no. That means it runs in the family!" Bad blood notwithstanding, I choose to believe that I've got juicy blood and that I will resist TB, heart attacks, et al and live to be a venerable old woman with a cane carved by a great African chieftain—like Ms. Margaret Mead.

Mary, the woman I work for, has zero breasts. . . . I had to type something for her and arrived at a section titled "Health," and there it was. The right one in 1960, the left—as a "preventive measure"—in 1967. Present health—"Excellent!" she shouts from the page.
God save my breasts.
(In a moment of black humor yesterday, I wondered if perhaps my boss had the second breast removed for the sake of symmetry.)

Interviewing for a television job. Judy, who I adore and who would be my boss, had a lumpectomy.
Can't escape the breast these days. . . .
Told Cathy I'm so traumatized I can't even react anymore.

_____

I was finding solace in my relationship with Meg. I was withdrawing my investment in my relationship with Philip. I didn't know that my sister was seeking some sort of solace for herself. Meg and I seemed to be staving off the world together. Doren, after years of hibernation, was now flinging herself into a world that was neither safe nor comforting.

I miss Candice terribly . . . which pretty much confirms my notion that more than sex right now, I am seeking some sort of communion. And I can't be more precise than that. Whatever it is, it is a communion I have been hungering after. It could have been with Candice if she had not decided to excavate in Greece.

Candice returns from her archaeological work this Christmas—briefly. I feel awfully glad about this and yet last Christmas was so difficult with her around. It appears that my idea of our relationship involves a great deal of fantasizing about the way I'd like it to be.

My comfort in the world continued to come in the form of women I could trust and depend on. That is where I felt safe. My friendships with women were nurturing, loving. It would take a long time to find those attributes in a relationship with a man. Doren felt with other women she had to tone down the person she was. She felt she was too overwhelming, too intense, her demeanor too threatening. Doren did not want to suppress the passionate side of her nature, and it seemed to her that passion and intensity were appropriate only within an intimate relationship with a man. I, on the other hand, had friendships with women that, along with the inherent safety, could reach levels of emotion that were just as powerful, albeit different, as the passion I would experience with a man.

I ran into Ashley—now married and big in the belly with child—today in Harvard Square. Why did she look wonderful to me? She has just missed having a miscarriage and is very white and scared and we were never friends, and yet . . . I hope I didn't scare her off by coming on so strong. "You look very good," I said. "So do you," she said, smiling just a little too brightly.

I miss Candice. And I know Ashley would be a substitute. But perhaps not a bad one. I fantasized in the subway that we would become fast friends and that I would love her baby, and that at least once a week I would say to Andrew, "I'm going over to Ashley's today to play with the baby."

I hope I didn't frighten Ashley. I really am looking forward to a good, long talk with her. Even if that's the beginning and end of it. . . . Funny that just a few minutes before I had seen a girl crossing the street and remarked to Andrew that from the back she looked just like Candice in the Bryn Mawr days. Thick blond hair loosely pinned up, pea coat, tight, faded jeans, Weejuns. Andrew agreed that the walk and build of the girl were both astonishingly reminiscent of Candice.

I'm going to call Ashley if she doesn't call me. I'm going to ask her when she'd like to visit. And what time is best for her. And what she'd like to eat or not eat.

Something in me feels like spring.
Pachelbel Canon in D Major on the stereo, the sun pouring into the apartment like some metaphoric, undeserved blessing. . . .
The faint stir of hope in my bones that something—something wonderful perhaps—may happen yet if only I forbear.

For the first time in my entire menstruating life, I got my period nearly ten days too soon. I was so frightened I called my mother right away to ascertain whether or not I had a right to be frightened.
She said that I did not.
She said only if it went on for "months" this way.
But underneath my placid—even contented—acceptance of this phenomenon lies a very deep and abiding fear that the fates will not permit me to live, will not permit me to be happy, for whatever the reasons, for whatever the time.

_____

Another anniversary is just a few days away. Four years since Doren has died. I hate the word "anniversary." Anniversary has celebratory connotations. Anniversary and death don't go together. The twenty-second of March dog-ears every year for me. How am I now? I ask myself. How is grief different now than last year, the year before, the year before that, and so on? This time I have had two preceding weeks of emotional turmoil. When friends ask casually how I am, I say, "I don't know. Teary. Weird. I don't know why." Then I start asking myself: Is this connected to the twenty-second? I don't want to believe it is. Last year didn't feel like this. It didn't feel as hard. Why is it this way now? Why did I cry myself to sleep last night? Why does this feel like abandonment, like a renewal of a despairing grief?

This time I am thirty-three. Thirty-three on March twenty-second. The same age Doren was when she died. At thirty-three, on March twenty-second, Doren's life was over. Mine is not. I am moving on. I am living. I am growing beyond my sister's years. After the twenty-second, I will be the older sister. There has been an impossible twist of nature. For the past two weeks I have been raging against it. As I felt defeated when Doren died, now I feel defeat in the fact that I go on living, without her. Beyond her.

It is 22 March 1985 and I feel as if I am passing through some godforsaken rite of passage into darkness. The day has me caught between worlds, and I can't name those worlds. What I'm going to say doesn't make sense, but why should it? I do want to live, but I do not want to live beyond Doren's years. I don't want this change. I'm afraid of it. This year, on this day, my sister's death, the fact of it, comes back to me full-force. I feel as if my grief has been split open. Inside there is a deafening sound.

Has my sister's spirit grown old with me, as she would have? Does it continue to age, as I do? I don't want to pass through the world without my older sister. I want, at least, her older spirit with me. I don't want to think of her young anymore, because now she will be younger than I am. But when I think of her at thirty-seven, which she would have been at this time had she lived, I begin to stumble because then I have to invent an entire life for her. Where would she have been now? What would have transpired in her life over the past four years had she survived in health? I can't give myself that task of invention. Because it would be just that. Invention. And it would be false.

Now I travel on, unprotected. No longer the younger sister. Since my sister's death I have been deferring, still, to the older sister's wisdom. And now my own experience will bring me wisdom that surpasses hers. Yet I insist on taking Doren with me. I cannot leave her behind. She must still teach me things.

I could barely wait to graduate from college. I came up with a plan that would declare my upcoming freedom— travel through Europe. That, in itself, was not a startling proposition. Everyone my age was doing it then. Backpacks were selling like crazy, along with "Let's Go! Europe!" guidebooks, along with student fares that would get you there and back for two hundred dollars. I would do something different. At least different from any of my female friends: I would travel alone.

My decision startled the people who knew me. Mostly, it shocked *me*. It threw my family into a tailspin. How could I possibly consider it? Although I reassured everyone I was perfectly capable of traveling alone, I didn't, in any way, convince myself. I was scared to death and I had no idea why I wanted to subject myself to such an unknown experience. I had countless nightmares. I imagined what it would feel like to be so far away from anyone I knew, to be so unprotected, to be so on my own. I was not at all excited, and yet I continued to follow through with my plans. When I saw that no one really believed I would, or could, do this, their disbelief began to serve as my impetus.

As I was planning my "break," so to speak, Doren was planning one too. She was not, however, talking about it.

Sitting in a playground, surrounded by frolicking children—just what I need. "Papa, wanna see how good I can ride?"

Is that all the world is doing—procreating? There's a nice-looking, mustached young man across the sandbox, tying shoelaces on a five-year-old girl. I'll never catch up with the so-called normal. Never.

And Andrew hates me for it because he is just about in step. A little off—but reasonably in step. PhD. achieved, he's ready for bigger money and babies. Why not? The pity (for him) is—he can't admit it as long as he's living (trying to live) with me.

We should not be together.

When will I face up to that off the printed page? Could I feel any more lonely than I do tonight? NO. So it must be the failure thing, the public admission: "I goofed."

And regret. And separation pains.

But the sooner begun, the better. Where could I start? New York would be hell—is there any other choice? Europe. London. It's a long shot, but worth considering.

New York would mean a good job and a lousy living situation—but . . . infinite people possibilities. Must think about it seriously.

"Wanna ride up the street?"

"No."

"Wanna take your bike home?"

"No!"

"Wanna go to sleep!"

"No, No, No!" The five-year-old breaks into tears.

Doren and I were both in New York during Christmas and New Year's 1972. Sometimes there would be two typewriters going at the same time. I brought mine from Boston and typed in our old bedroom. Doren used George's typewriter and typed in the living room. I was more threatened by this than comforted.

I just moved Doren's suitcase and other scattered belongings into the dining room. I don't want her things in here. I need some privacy. I've gotten lost in the chaos of family. It is 10 P.M. and everyone is going to sleep. I cannot. Someone will probably stop me from typing. Doren just walked in, then turned her back and shut the door. Now she is screaming. At Andrew? Or about me? I can't stand this. I need OUT! Stuffed a blanket under the typewriter to muffle the sound. Jesus, this typing is loud. Waiting for Doren to walk in and silence me. . . . Earlier, Andrew walked in. I put my hand up as a stop sign, so he does not come near my journal page. "You're just like Doren," he says laughing, and hugs me. He eases his way out of my room. Then Doren appears. "You're typing?" Another nod from here at the typewriter. She waves and exits. She knows.

Although my mother and I had had a conversation in which she told me she accepted me as a writer, if that's what I decided to be, I didn't believe her. This didn't mean, she said, that I would sit down and write books like Doren. I could be a writer of television, movies, an editor, she suggested. I informed her I was not going to retreat from my writing just because Doren also writes. I am separate from her, I claimed. My mother agreed that I was, but her concern did not seem to diminish.

During that Christmas vacation my best source of support came from Meg, who was driving south and stopping to call me along the way. I was turning to Meg for the support I had been used to receiving from my sister.

Meg called from Atlanta. She heard me last night, she says. She heard my spirit yelling. She knew she had to call. I'm straining so hard to reach her, straining to hear her over the static. I want to catch every word, every mood. She can hear me fine, she says.

I knew Doren was moving further away from her marriage, and I was angry. We didn't talk about it. An interesting event occurred that Christmas of '72. It was a repeat performance. I arrived home one day, eager to pounce on my typewriter, and entered my New York bedroom—and, as I had witnessed many years before, it had been rearranged. Doren had been seized again with the desire to send me a sibling message via this room. It was another apex of our competitiveness and hostility toward one another. The ironic part was that neither of us actually lived in this room anymore, and yet we both still meant to claim it.

Did I mention that I spent half the day doing over Cathy's room?
Well, it isn't Cathy's room anymore. She has to know that I have just as much right to be comfortable when I visit as she does.

And now that she has her own apartment, I think it's fair I did what I did—leaving much of the material intact and placed as she wished. It's not pretty, but it's now functional.

Competition aside, and it did seem that it was possible to put it aside, Doren was clearly under a great deal of stress and I remained concerned about her. Because she wouldn't tell me the nuances of her life and emotions then, there seemed little I could do in the way of comfort. Even so, she offered some comfort of her own. It came by way of a postcard when we were both in Boston. She could have, just as easily, relayed her message over the phone. I don't think it is insignificant that the painting on the card, called *Fair Girl with a Doll*, by August Macke, looks to me like a young girl sitting on a chair with a younger girl on her lap. The younger girl, the doll, could be her little sister. And the older sister is smiling almost imperceptibly, but smiling nonetheless.

Dear Cathy—

The hollow tone of my voice to the contrary, your calls—and, even more important—your faith and love *are* helping. A lot.

Love,
Grateful Sister

Although there was unspoken drama continuing to unfold in my sister's life, things seemed to proceed as usual in Boston. I continued to spend time with Doren and Andrew. I was still hoping their relationship would subsist, although if pressed for an opinion, I don't think I believed it was thriving.

As charmed as I was with Meg, my emotions did a turnaround by the end of senior year. It was a surprise to me, and more to her, that I felt as if I hated her. I simply no longer wanted her around. I thought Meg was trying to take something away from me. It irked me that, admiring my hiking boots, she bought the same pair. Admiring my writing, she wrote stories incorporating some of my own lines. I didn't believe her that this was inadvertent. I thought she was robbing me of my very identity. I couldn't explain any of this to her. I just suddenly, and without explanation, withdrew from our relationship. Meg was clearly distraught, but this didn't affect me except to make me more uncomfortable, more intolerant. She told me she loved me. I turned my emotions to ice. I never had to cope with any feelings of separation when June hit. It was going to be a clean and acceptable break, with nothing to wrench me off my chosen track.

> Four years of Boston—OVER. Twenty-one years of school—OVER. Most relationships materialized over the past four years—OVER. What is it I take with me? Most important—my relationship with my sister that might never have been had I not lived close to her these past four years. She has contributed her soul to my life. . . . Trying to 'camouflage endings with thoughts of continuance so that I walk out of this apartment door, steady.

Dear Candice—

. . . I need to begin again and I don't know how to begin again, given the enormous commitment I made to Andrew several (almost five) years ago. It defies reason, Candice, the way I am suffering now; the prison I feel myself to be in. And the prison composed simply of compromises—mostly small ones, even. I am daily beaten by circumstances I helped create. And I want to destroy them and start fresh—if that is possible—but everything is against it. Everything. Even my family and few friends—including you—who clearly see that Andrew is a good and an honorable man, but fail to see, or choose not to notice, that the bond between us is absolutely killing me.

. . . I miss—have been missing for some time—having you to talk to. . . .

There were no emotional good-byes between my sister and me upon my departure from Boston. I didn't feel I was leaving her behind. I was unaware, however, that before the end of the year, we would be together again, living, still, in the same city, independent women pursuing our careers. Doren followed me to New York, leaving behind everything in Boston except her relationship with her sister, the only relationship in our lives that brought us comfort and stability because, in its stubbornness, agility, and irrationality, it defied separation.

13

Candice comes to New York to visit. I have seen her only a couple of times since Doren died. The last time, about two years ago, she was here with her husband, Scott. I joined them at the Metropolitan Museum of Art. Candice was brimming with knowledge and explained everything to me with clarity and creativity. She was teaching me things, just as she had for Doren. This must be how Doren felt, I thought, as Candice talked to me about the figures on an ancient sarcophagus. I could almost imagine the hands of the artist carving out the myths. Scott spoke softly, taking me over to his favorite tapestry, teaching me what all those horses and riders and castles mean. Four years ago I saw them on their Virginia farm. That's when we buried the ashes on the promontory. Now, Candice sits in my apartment and as she talks I hear Doren's voice, I can feel Doren's affection for her closest friend, I imagine them talking intimately as Doren has described in her journal. This woman was Doren's closest friend. Now she is the closest I get to Doren. Candice is losing faith that I will ever return to the farm. For four years I have had excuses. None of them tell the real reason. The truth is that I know it is where I will feel Doren's presence the most, and her absence.

I walk into Doren's apartment on Tenth Street and I am safe. I am breathless from six flights of stairs and she is waiting at the door holding out to me a glass of juice and seltzer. I take the glass, nodding gratefully, and walk into the narrow hallway as she closes the door behind us, sliding the police-lock bar into position. Then I get a hug. Enfolded by her arms, held close to the warmth of my sister's body, is where I'd like to be more than any other place in the world at that moment. I have taken the subway down to where she lives to get a dose of comfort. The man I love is not loving me. The man Doren loves is not loving her.

Alone we cry. Together we laugh. We find our humor, we find what we respect in ourselves. Doren puts out a platter of cherry tomatoes, kirby cucumbers, swiss cheese, caviar, crackers that are salty and crackers that are sweet. We sit on her couch, she has a shawl around her shoulders and she has given me a plaid afghan to curl up under, and we talk and laugh and gesture for hours. Then she plays me a forty-five record she has fallen in love with and bought that week. "Shoo-rah! Shoo-rah! I can see you comin' / Shoo-rah! Shoo-rah! but you won't catch me!" Before I leave she gives me the record because I love it as much as she does and she has been playing it, anyway, for days. "And now," she says, "it's yours."

*B*efore moving to New York permanently, Doren was traveling back and forth from Boston. I returned to my mother's home before going to Europe the summer after graduating from Boston University. Doren was convincing herself to leave Andrew; she was telling me she had never loved Andrew at all. I had little patience with her. I didn't believe her. I never believed this. It was a claim Doren never withdrew. It was a claim I continued to protest. She convinced everyone who knew her, my parents included, that what appeared to be love for Andrew was not. There was nothing to argue, I said. I told my parents, and I told my sister, "I happen to know. I was there."

It was difficult to be supportive of my sister when she was in such a tailspin. She appeared to be manic, but I wasn't aware of how distraught and disoriented she was. I wasn't aware of what can happen at the end of a marriage, how divorce has the power to transform self-respect into a demon hate. Doren was flinging herself onto the world with a vengeance, and I couldn't watch from the front row.

Candice—

Do you know what a nervous breakdown is?? Well, I had one and am still kind of reeling from the shock and pain. One of the things is that one does not function at one's peak—in fact one barely *functions at all.* . . .

I can't talk about Andrew yet—too scary and horrible. . . . I was provoked beyond human endurance. . . . Andrew and I are going to be divorced. *It must be*. Explanations later when my stomach hurts less.

Please be my friend. Patience! Write again and next time I will send a *lot more*. I am still *your* friend.

Love, Doren

. . . The other afternoon I don't know what possessed me but I felt "clean" and free of my own past, and so I went into what was once my sister's closet in my mother's house and took out my wedding dress (it has been stored in there since the day of the wedding). . . . Anyway, I had been working on a job tryout and I was dirty and sweaty from head to foot, but I took my beautiful Mexican wedding dress and the beautiful white satin slip that I had had custom-made and I put them both on. And, dirty and unkempt as I was, I looked in a full mirror at myself and had to start smiling. . . . I looked beautiful! What a shock! I have looked so ugly to myself for the last five (or is it six?) years. . . . I felt beautiful the summer before I met Andrew. . . . During the years with him I looked at myself in the mirror and couldn't recognize my own face. . . . I had planned the dress to be reusable, yet the wedding was such an agony, and the realization that I was wedding the wrong man hit me so hard the night I married, I entrusted the dress tearfully to Cathy that night . . . told her then, and many times later, that I didn't want to throw it away, but that I doubted I would ever be able to wear it again. . . .

Doren was compelled to wipe Andrew off the face of the earth, scrub her emotions clean of him. It seemed as though it was the only way she could cope with the divorce, with what she felt was a personal failure. "I never loved him anyway" was easier than "I loved him and it didn't work and I am in pain."

My Europe plans held fast. As the 747 lifted off the ground I felt a rush of enormous relief. Leaving New York. Leaving my family. My friends. I was on my own, responsible only to myself. I felt soothed. This surprised me. The calm was unexpected. I was on my way to Europe, alone, and I was euphoric.

Everywhere I traveled I felt a kinship with "place," with history. I touched every piece of marble and stone the signs instructed me not to. I wanted the history to seep into my body, to stay with me, to always keep me feeling so peaceful, so grounded, so much a part of a whole. It was as if my life had meaning for the first time, standing in a place that had existed for thousands of years. I felt I belonged. With my red backpack, my hiking boots, my army pants, my T-shirts, I wandered through Holland and France and Switzerland and Italy and Greece and England with a tear-drenched map. I was overwhelmed by all the beauty. All the while I kept a journal and sent postcards and aerograms home.

Dearest Cookie—Will you still love us when you return, sophisticated lady?

I traveled through Europe, out of sync with the child's helplessness I had grown accustomed to. When I returned to New York in the fall, I needed a job. Initially utilizing my mother's connections, Doren and I both began working at New York publishing companies. My mother had, in the ten years since she had entered the business world, become a publishing executive. Neither Doren nor I felt we were following in her footsteps. We saw ourselves as writers first, and so needed a way to make a living. At that time the nine-to-five method was all I knew, and although I functioned well with office work and office politics and banal elevator dialogue, I felt a discomfort with it all. However, working in an office was the only way to be an adult, I thought, so I kept on. At least for a while.

Doren had a harder time with office life. Her exuberance, enthusiasm, intelligence, and efficiency burst from her in ways which sometimes alienated people. Doren "came on strong." She *tried* so hard, feeling pressured, as always, to excel. Office politics left Doren baffled. She didn't know about being discreet regarding your own cleverness around people who might resent you for it. The saying in my family had always been that Cathy was the one with common sense and Doren was the one without any.

Even though we were at different levels of personal experience, we bore a striking resemblance when it came to selfdoubt and insecurity. This went hand in hand with similar grandiose notions about ourselves. We thought we were the best and we thought we were the worst. Sometimes we seemed to be the same person.

Christ, still I am waiting. At my desk waiting. No matter who it is, I am always having to wait.

Why do I always find myself waiting? And when will I learn to do it gracefully?

Doren moved into an apartment in Greenwich Village. It wasn't any old apartment. It was our father's. He had rented it for years, even when he and my mother were still married. Then he lived there, for a very short time, after their divorce. Now Doren was getting it for peanuts. I didn't want it, not even for peanuts. I still thought of my father as one of the untouchables, a man whose life I refused to allow to touch mine. I may have been trying to be an adult in the business world, but I had no inclination to rise to that status in my relationship with my father. Doren, frankly, thought I was an idiot not to want the apartment and to let her have it without a fuss. I had other intentions. I moved to an Upper West Side apartment, five blocks away from my mother. This, I thought, was sane.

Candice—

O.K. I'm put back together again, somewhat—laboring on "new" apt. (in the *Village* of all places), trying to get through the bitterest stuff with Andrew (*divorce* is what *he* wants and now I do too) . . . but what a terrible mess it is. . . . By Xmas I *should* be a *wonderful, new,* and *independent woman!* . . .

Candice—

. . . Flew to Cambridge on Monday (a day that will live in infamy) at 7:00 A.M. to get divorced. Without question one of the 5 worst days of my life. Let it suffice (for now) that it ain't like *Perry Mason* . . . and telling the sad tale of my last day with Andrew in front of judge and *packed* audience (gallery?) was teeth-and-knee-rocking . . . and worse, worse, worse. . . . Flew back, though, to NYC at 11:00 A.M., got into bed, "pretended" sickness, and re-covered by 8:00 P.M. I was "me" again.

I was living alone in the neighborhood of my adolescence. I loved my apartment, but I didn't love the ghosts. Walking around outside, I'd pass all the landmarks from the latter part of my childhood. I'd feel the old feelings. The park benches across the street from Walden, where we'd go for cigarette breaks; the drugstore that no longer had the soda fountain where I used to hang out after school; the pizza parlor that replaced the drugstore when the soda fountain was taken out; the building I lived in with my mother, my father, and Doren, then my mother and father, then my mother, where now my mother lived with George. Taking a walk was no mere stroll. Although I was happy in my new apartment and proud to be among those in the world who worked to make a living, I felt raw. I didn't like the feeling, and I searched for methods to feel more in control.

I want to be honest now—so much so that I will cry even if I am angry at myself for crying because *I like the raw*—it is part of who I am, and it is part of my new strength . . . because if I stay true to the "raw" (i.e., my instinctive self) I will know—instinctively—what to do now—step by step. . . .

Because Doren felt she had been numb throughout her marriage, being raw was a preferred alternative. For me it was no alternative at all. There was just so much I could take of my own vulnerability. If I had to be vulnerable, I thought, I may as well put it to good use. The only good use I knew of was to filter it through my creative resources. I began taking guitar lessons, I bought reams of classical piano music and played Bach and Mozart daily on the piano from my childhood, now in my own apartment, and I began to write poems. I was most content, most euphoric, when I was alone with my guitar, piano, or typewriter. I could depend on them. They were consistent. I was learning to nurture myself outside a relationship with a man.

I moved around between publishing companies, working first in editorial departments, then in publicity. This life seemed reasonable, even fun, until my writing started to take precedence. The editor of a literary magazine had seen my poems and invited me, on scholarship, to a writers' conference sponsored by the magazine. This was my first, tangible recognition from the "real" world. It wasn't from Doren, it wasn't from a professor. But this was also a wrench thrown into my relationship with my sister. I was getting recognition as a writer before Doren. That wasn't supposed to happen. Family myths are obstinate. Doren was still the writer; I was still supposed to be the actress.

————————

My only option is to write something fine. What I will try to do, perhaps, starting tomorrow is to get going with my writing. . . . Otherwise I will feel doomed. . . .

Dear Candice—

I have (wisely? unwisely?) left publishing for a spell to try to write. . . .

————————

I did the same.

1974. Doren and Andrew are no longer together, but where does it say that I have to lose Andrew? We arrange to go mountain climbing together in late August. I will take a train to Cambridge, stay with Andrew, and drive with him to the White Mountains in New Hampshire. Where Doren and I used to climb at Trebor.

Andrew still lives in the same house. It seems as if sun no longer enters here. Nothing looks the same. He has turned the bedroom into his office. He sleeps on the living room floor. Even the furniture, what is left of it, is dark, old wood. There is no color anywhere. Doren isn't anywhere. I keep looking for Doren in this house. Andrew keeps smiling, but I don't buy his joviality for a minute. I am glad when we leave in the morning for New Hampshire. Andrew and I climb the mountain through rain and thick mist. After a few hours we reach the AMC hut where we stay for the night. I am happy to be with him, but it is awkward. Something is so obviously missing. Our relationship is no longer safe, no longer defined. The next day includes rock climbing in order to reach the summit. We are climbing against 50 mph winds, 12° wind-chill factor. At one point I am so literally paralyzed with fear, my feet refuse to move. Andrew is above me, reaching for me, asking me to trust him, to trust myself, to move my foot to the next small ledge. He promises me I will be all right. He promises. I don't know how my foot moves, but it does. I join him at the top and there is a 360° view. The wind is still icy and strong. I realize it is not written anywhere that I must lose Andrew, but I know I will lose him. He knows it too. I can tell. He has known it for a while now.

1974. Doren and I talk nonstop on the train ride to and from East Hampton. We talk nonstop at Mother's house. We giggle late at night in our twin beds in the guest room. It feels so much like when we were children I am surprised we don't play tent. We lie on the beach at the bay and hate the flies together. We gossip about anything we can think of, even Mother and George when they are not within earshot. We go with them to a party and sit together on a couch, and talk. I notice we are looking at the same attractive man. Doren gets up to talk to him before I do. I notice we don't acknowledge this. We talk incessantly on the train ride back to the city, and comment on the Fellini types riding on the train. We listen to other people's conversations and exchange knowing glances. We play the story game on a legal pad. Doren writes a sentence, folds it so I can't see it, then I write a sentence under that, fold it so she can't see it, and so on. The point is to see how mystically attuned we are to one another. We conclude we are very mystically attuned.

DOREN: Pale blue, navy blue, bright blue, gray blue . . .

CATHY: When I relax I will feel as good as the porcelain rabbit; sprout green leaves . . .

DOREN: Sorrow pouring from her fingers like honey. Like milk.

CATHY: Every night I would like to look up and see that starburst.

DOREN: (On days like this I would take nine or ten baths.)

CATHY: The typewriter keys are exacting; I am freed.

DOREN: (. . . Or invite my Lithuanian masseuse over . . .)

CATHY: You are more than just a comfort.

DOREN: Water with you is more than water. Grief, more than grief.

CATHY: Better thoughts: the night you stayed up with me during a thunderstorm, sat at the edge of my bed, held my feet.

DOREN: Now I see orange. Fruit. Sun.

CATHY: Do you know that the huge, spread-eagled plant on my piano is dependent on me for survival?

DOREN: "My sister," she said huskily, "is the salt of the earth."

*D*oren stopped working nine-to-five so that she could try to write. She made a living doing various forms of free-lance writing. Some of it came from me, through the company I was with. I had wanted to help Doren and later realized I was not helping myself. I was giving her work that would otherwise have been assigned to me. The biggest problem came when I gave up the nine-to-five route as well. Then we were obviously competing for the same free-lance jobs. When it came down to who would go after which job, if Doren wanted what I wanted, I conceded. I thought she had more right to it than I. She had been around longer. She had more experience. She was the older sister. She deserved it. I, on the other hand, didn't expect very much for myself. When something came through that I wanted, and worked for, it still seemed to elude me.

I was beginning to write book reviews, publish poetry, and still my achievements seemed unreal to me. No matter what I accomplished in my work, I thought of myself as unproductive.

. . . After turning down a few pretty good jobs, I decided to stop for a bit in order to think about whether or not I'd like to be a free-lance journalist, manuscript reader, and/or other part-time things while I try to write. . . . I have begun—quite mysteriously—to think of myself as a writer, which amuses me greatly when I consider that for years I have listened to other people tell me I am a writer while thinking always, "A lot YOU know!" . . .

. . . I am working on my head—trying to empty it of men—so that I can write. It feels like my brains are infested.

I can be a writer if I can hold on to my rage and my joy. . . .

Endings are not altogether different from beginnings—one's flesh prickles, one shivers, one feels excited and afraid. The only difference is that beginnings have everything to do with hope, and endings are associated with despair.

After returning from the writers' conference, I began writing every day. It was during the summer of 1975, the heat and flies gathered around the ceiling light in the living room during the day, the street noises clanked in through the wide-open windows. Sweating from the heat, and taking a few showers a day were the prerequisites for writing poems. By the end of the summer I sat down one morning to write another one and I knew I had something else on my hands. I told myself to stop breaking up the lines. I was writing longhand, as was customary for poems, and suddenly I found myself at the typewriter. I turned the stanzas into sentences, paragraphs, pages. By the afternoon I had the beginning of a novel. Within weeks I gave notice at my job. "I'm writing a novel," I told everyone. I was changing my entire life because of ten pages. I thought I was out of my mind, but I accepted that predicament.

The days were mine. I didn't have to be anywhere except where I wanted to be. In those first months, waking up every day and going right to my typewriter, I felt I was harboring a deep and wondrous secret. I was doing in the world exactly what I wanted to be doing. How was this possible? I thought. I had no idea how I would make a living, but I didn't have a problem getting enough free-lance writing to survive. I had all I needed: My apartment, food, a typewriter. My book.

My old friend Emily was also living in New York, pursuing an acting career. She was crucial to the writing of my novel, listening to me read chapters aloud week by week, and helping me edit. We would have late-night work sessions that would segue into dialogues about lost, and found, love. Emily had just found. She was seeing a man and falling in love. I wasn't jealous—I was writing.

The content of my novel began to disturb me. It was somber. My darkness was emerging, not the joy. I thought, perhaps, that I was involved in an exorcism. In order to write the book, I was thinking in fatalistic terms, I was dwelling on tragedy and death. The main character angered me with her dark notions of life, and yet she was so familiar to me, so close.

. . . The pain just seems to deepen. . . . It's terrible this beginning again. More lonely than death. And more terrible than the grief of loss is the grief of pure and total emptiness. . . . Grief, after all, is circular. It turns back and back upon itself and there is no way out—just around and around. . . .

. . . Cathy has been tremendously comforting—always there with the right words at the right time. . . . She heard me saying over and over that I felt confused and she said finally, "You are not confused. You know exactly what you feel and what you want to do." And she was on target. I did.

When I felt the most despair I put my arms around my typewriter, put my head down on it, and wept. "This is all I have," I would say aloud.

When I finished the novel I was euphoric for as long as it took to call everyone I knew to tell them I had completed my book. Then the shock set in. When I awoke the next morning I no longer had my book to turn to. I had been doing in the world what I most wanted to do, and suddenly it was no longer there for me. I hadn't expected or anticipated this change.

I was not in good shape. I left town, visiting an old friend out West. I spent my days either sitting in a small park or sitting in my friend's living room staring at walls. She went to work every day, so I was left to my own devices. My devices were nil.

When I returned to New York, Doren was concerned that I was so out of sorts. She was involved in a poetry-writing workshop that met once a week at various people's homes. She offered to take me to one of the workshops. We coped with our competition vis-à-vis work by fudging boundaries. As I had invited Doren into my class with John Barth, she was inviting me into her writing workshop as well. Anything short of sharing what was important to us produced instantaneous guilt.

In Doren's poetry workshop she met Isshin. Isshin was Japanese, he practiced Zen, he was a poet, he was peaceful. Doren was drawn to that peace.

Children.
One man. One man for a long time. (Frightening.)
Career. (Frightening and exciting.)
Confessions: I think he loves me and it makes me feel good, but not the way I expected to feel—this time, this at-last time. . . . Mostly I think of my children. . . . Is this the moment? I think. . . . I really think this is the moment, and I know there is no one—not one single person who would agree, or at least understand my romanticism. . . . Isshin wants to take a course in "intimate relationships" at the New School . . . happiness/misery quotients and

all. . . . I laughed more than I let myself show. . . . Isshin. He is certainly a departure. . . . in that he reminds me—in significant ways—of myself. Considerate, sensual, direct, etc. Non-macho man. God, what a pleasure. . . . But how it reminds me of my rage against others. . . .

What next? What nest next?

————————

Doren went back to work. Now she was in the movie business, working as Story Editor for a small film company. I continued to free-lance. Making a living in this way was difficult, but I liked having the freedom to shape my days. My days, however, became increasingly tension-filled. I missed writing the novel. Like many first novels, it met its fate in the back of an already overstuffed filing cabinet. I felt so isolated, and on one very hot day in August of 1976 I thought I was losing my mind. August is a very bad time in New York to feel like you're losing your mind. Psychiatrists vacation in August. I managed to find one of the few therapists left in town and I began to discover that my sorrow had been years in the making. This was the same therapist who, a few years later, would hold me in her arms as I shrieked and sobbed, curling myself into the tightest fetal position imaginable after receiving the news that Doren's breast cancer had spread to her liver, lungs, and brain.

During the summer that I believed myself to be on the wrong side of reality, I spent weekends at my mother and George's house in East Hampton, in the company and comfort of them and Doren and Isshin. I felt warm toward Isshin but I did not allow myself to adopt him as I had Andrew. Isshin taught me Zen meditation. His kindness was clear, without ornament. Doren and I were amazed at how he could "sit" for hours, his feet turning blue. We admired his patience, his calm, his spirit, which seemed to carry him through the world without fearing harm. On occasion Isshin joined Doren and me in our story game. When the folded paper came around to him, he always looked amused. He always blushed.

> ISSHIN: Especially two beautiful sisters looked at each other. I smiled.
> CATHY: . . . on his sled; down the hill in December . . .
> DOREN: . . . and then I felt very sick to my stomach and . . .
> ISSHIN: Oops, pits came out and luxurious scent of magnolia . . .

CATHY: Grating, so grating it compares to the subway din, and my ears . . .

DOREN: . . . because I love Isshin!

ISSHIN: Her heart throbbed as the watermelon appeared . . .

CATHY: I would never, *never* pose by a gravestone . . .

DOREN: . . . with trees in my hair . . .

ISSHIN: . . . and sometimes it's a bunch of dried twigs on the ground . . .

I don't recall confiding to any of my friends the extent of my distress. They knew I was not at my best, but I hadn't found the vocabulary to describe what I was feeling. I felt I was putting on a good normality show for everyone. I was functioning, working, carrying on conversations without anyone discerning that I was in absentia.

It was during this time that my friend Emily announced she was going to marry. The shock of this was so great for me, I could barely dredge up excitement for her. Emily was the devout feminist, the devout Marxist, the devout actress. Was she now going to be a devout wife? I went to her wedding and cried from beginning to end. Emily was now set apart from her group of friends. She had a ring on her finger and a man permanently in her bed. We did not.

There was also the reappearance of Meg. The woman I had virtually abandoned. I had met someone at the writers' conference who knew her. I was curious about what Meg was doing in her life now and heard she was still living in Boston, had written a novel, and was writing book reviews. As an aside, I heard mention of Meg's lover, and the pronoun used was feminine. "Excuse me," I said, quietly and trembling, "could you repeat what you just said?" Again, the *she* word. "Meg is with a woman?" I inquired, my voice up an octave or two. "Oh yes," I was told, quite matter-of-factly. "Meg is gay, didn't you know that?" The news sent me reeling.

Meg called me not too long after that. She had heard I was at the conference. She was going to be in New York for a weekend and wanted to see me. Meg sat in my apartment and told me she had thought all these years that I had known she was gay. She thought I knew she was in love with me, and that that was why I had rejected her so completely. "I had no idea," I kept saying to her that afternoon. I had no idea, I had no idea. During our senior year at college, as I was withdrawing from our friendship, Meg had her first lesbian relationship.

Although she had never told me about it, she had convinced herself I must have known.

The news, although at first startling, also brought relief. It didn't just explain Meg to me, it was a piece, albeit vague, about myself that would later bring to light the substance of all my relationships—my quest for, and unconscious rejection of, intimacy.

Doren emerges as the pulse of that heart.

I've been avoiding Doren like the plague. She's taken up with someone new. Isshin is out. Rob is in. She says she is in love. I don't even want to hear it. She says he is the man of her life. She's known him only a few weeks, and he is living with someone else to boot. He is about to move in with Doren. It is too fast, too desperate for my taste. I don't trust it. Love, love, love, want, want, want, now, now, now, need, need, need. No siree, don't trust it at all. I'm not exactly a foreigner on this terrain. I'd like to isolate myself from all this. I'd like to live in the mountains.

I've been avoiding Doren like the plague. It has been months since her breast cancer, months since I told her I needed to be on my own for a while. Months since I first made an attempt to live my life without familial intrusions. Without Doren's opinion. How can I know my own opinion when Doren is always hanging around? On my way to see someone in the Village, I see Doren walking toward me. I bump into my own sister on the street as if we are casual acquaintances. It is a spring day. Neither of us is wearing a coat. Doren is wearing bright colors. Her hair is bouncing. She is smiling. We don't hug. I know she is happier to see me than I am to see her. She looks beautiful. I don't tell her that.

Doren received word from Andrew that he was planning to marry. He needed her help. The woman he was marrying was Catholic and in order for the Catholic Church to honor the marriage, Doren and Andrew's marriage would have to be rendered null and void. After much deliberation Doren finally decided she could not take part in the procedure.

Dear Rev. Peters:

My phone conversation with you last week has caused me tremendous anguish. Though I had wanted to cooperate in this procedure for Andrew's sake, many days of soul-searching have brought me to a different understanding of the situation. My conscience does not allow me to participate in this ceremony, which seems to me to betray not only my deep feelings about my Jewishness, but also about my own marriage, now dissolved. Affirming the fact that neither Andrew nor I have been baptized would assist the Church in declaring our marriage never existed in the eyes of God. I simply can't accept being part of this un-writing of history.

I also want to say without personal rancor that involving an ex-spouse in this manner is rather medieval and potentially harmful to all parties. I hope that in the future it will not be necessary.

Dear Andrew:

Though I did talk to Rev. Peters on the telephone, it caused me tremendous anguish. After many days of soul-searching I have decided to follow my conscience and not participate in this procedure. Please understand that this decision arises not out of any rancor—simply from my own, deep moral feelings about myself and my Jewishness. Your decision to honor the Catholic Church in a ceremonial—or any other—way is yours. Mine not to honor it must be considered equally legitimate.

I have returned the questionnaire, unsigned, to Rev. Peters with a personal note similar to this one. I regret having promised to do something which in the end I could not do, but I know you never wanted me to do that which I found morally impossible.

Doren was giving up the peace she had with Isshin. She was returning to another kind of passion, and for her it was a return to agony. Passion and agony, she thought, were necessarily linked and she knew no way around that dangerous coupling.

. . . As I get further away from adolescence, I see desire looming larger and larger. For me desire is not only large—it is a virtual centerpiece. Only thing bigger is death, or, as I like to think of it —fear of evaporation.

I keep wanting to be able to shine whether or not there is someone there to see me. But I can't. This thought is the worst. *I don't want to shine if no one will love me.*

Cathy called today to say that she likes Rob very much (we all spent some very relaxed time together last night) and that made me very happy indeed.

Doren and I were two independent women pursuing careers and yet we barely even noticed that part of ourselves. We were intelligent, attractive women only in the eyes of others. In our own eyes, we were needy, insecure, a couple of Poor Pitiful Pearls.

Love. We plunged toward the target like speeding trains. But the target was far away, unfocused. We weren't aware yet that love had to come from the inside out. What were we trying to grab hold of? A love that would fasten us to the earth, hold us immutable. We didn't know that love meant change. We were most compelled to draw consistency out of those who were most inconsistent.

Dear Candice—

Ready for large news? It's re love. Isshin and I separated . . . and . . . I met Rob—who is for the moment living at my house. . . . Rob, naturally, is terrific—and a far better mate for me than Andrew. He's a painter, by the way . . . 41, married before, no children, very tall and dark. . . . I don't know, I think I'm still looking at him cross-eyed with excitement. Yes, it does all seem terribly fast. . . . Anyway, I'm quite certain he is someone I can be with for a long time and I hope this wonderful feeling we have for each other is going to continue to grow despite the turmoil and dangers of ordinary life in N.Y.C. . . . or anywhere.

There are some new job possibilities, but, since the advent of Rob, I don't believe I'm at all keen to go to L.A., where some of the job prospects are. . . . We'll see. Truthfully, I'm going to be having a hell of a time this year resisting the desire to have a baby. Passion vs. profession! Jesus Christ.

Rob and Doren were not at all alike. I wanted to like him, for Doren's sake and for my own as well, since she brought him around a lot. But I couldn't muster enthusiasm about her relationship. Rob and I not only had nothing to say to each other, it seemed as if he had nothing to say at all. He was an artist and the first nonverbal man Doren had ever been with. Our mother seemed more upset by this than anyone. She had adored Isshin and now Doren was wanting her to adore a man who was, at best, aloof. When he and Doren were in the presence of others, they behaved as if they were not. Doren paid a lot of attention to Rob, but I was not confident he shared her abiding interest. I could never have imagined that Rob and I would spend endless hours together, a couple of years later, sitting in a hospital room, silent except for the sound of Doren's moist breathing.

Sometimes I feel broken in a way that can never be repaired. No amount of love, no degree of tenderness will ever add up to enough glue. . . .Time either sits heavy or darts like arrows in random flight. . . .

When I first really came to know Rob, the two of us on opposite sides of Doren's hospital bed, I grew less puzzled about what had brought them together. I felt their connection, and I wondered whether fate had played a part, given Doren's dying, given Rob's sitting with her day after day after day, his presence in her life so concentrated during those last months, his presence in her life at the moment of her death. Whatever turmoil had existed in their relationship, I witnessed a deep loyalty and commitment between them at the end that had nothing to do with convention.

I fear only what the fates can do—illness, death. I fear death in a way that is utterly different from anything I have ever experienced. But not tonight. I comfort myself with the feeling that my grandfather will watch over us until (at least) the birth of our first child. Yes, I do believe that.

Doren did become pregnant. But she never had the child she had waited so long for. This, above all else, more than the cancer that later invaded her body and eventually took her life, was, to Doren, her deepest tragedy. She had become pregnant accidentally, had wanted to carry through with the pregnancy, and Rob was opposed to the idea. This pregnancy was more important to Doren than anything that had come before. There wasn't any conceivable way she could have the child on her own. She would need Rob's support, both emotionally and financially. Most important, Doren wanted her child to have a father who would be present and available in that child's life. Rob would not make this commitment. Doren reluctantly chose to have an abortion.

My mother and I went with Doren to the clinic. We sat for hours in the waiting room. Neither of us spoke. The enormous sorrow of this event was clear. When Doren came out to us, the silence continued. We all walked down the street, Doren between us, her arms linked with ours. She was swallowing a lot, refusing to cry. She stopped at a phone booth to call Rob, to tell him she was all right. She felt she had to protect him, protect their relationship from her grief.

On July 21, 1978—last Friday—I had an abortion. I feel afraid right now that I will never forgive myself.

Rob is still here; since he didn't want our child, I don't really know why I still (think I) want him.

This grief makes all previous griefs seem small. I can't believe I swept my own child out of my body. I can't believe it.

The realization—when it hits (and I push it away as much as possible)—is so painful it feels like I won't be able to carry on living. Maybe I will; right now I wonder if life is worth *this*.

When Doren was experiencing her most awful sadness, I was in the midst of celebration. During the same month Doren became pregnant, I met Jeffrey, a film director. I felt that, finally, this was the relationship that would last me forever. There was passion combined with friendship, a new experience for me. My celebration became caught up in my sister's agony. That pattern would continue. My relationship with Jeffrey would be permanently affected by Doren's tragedy, by the tragedy that would become my own. Jeffrey and Doren became fused in my psyche. My love for my sister, and my anger toward her, for being ill, found another outlet. It was difficult, and ultimately impossible, to separate my feelings for these two people. Jeffrey had his own difficulties and fears, regarding not only his relationship with me but a troubled history that included a mother who had died of cancer. As deeply compelled as we were by one another, the combination was explosive. We struggled with and against each other for years, most of that time was during Doren's illness, and when our relationship finally ended, my anger never did. I could never blame my sister for dying, for leaving me. But I could blame Jeffrey for his weaknesses, for what I felt was his lack of courage.

Jeffrey and I are incredibly good together, comfortable, excited. Surely we are from the same litter. My smile muscles start to ache when I'm with him. But Doren had an abortion last Friday and she's struggling in the depths. And so the part of my life and myself that is Doren is grappling with her pain, and I am trying to help in any way I can. There are moments that stretch out when her pain becomes mine. I must learn how not to do that. I must learn to love without taking on someone else's pain.

I feel I have been living a total nightmare since the day I discovered I was pregnant. Why do I want to love him *still?* Why am I so afraid to let go of someone who gives me no place in his life? Why am I willing to settle for so little of what I need? . . . My life means absolutely nothing to me. I feel I am holding on to it, trying to make something better because the people outside expect me to. I expect so much misery to come, so much torment, so much disappointment, loss. . . . I get the job, I live alone. (I have the love, I lose the baby.) I feel like a juggler whose props are always smashing on the floor. Once in a while a few pieces float in the air. I smile; they crash.

I am broken. I am violated.

Because of Doren's abortion, her depression that followed, and the cancer appearing inside her six months later, one might assume a correlation between these events. The assumption is punishing to the one who is ill. I found support in not blaming my sister for her illness in Susan Sontag's crucial essay, "Illness as Metaphor." Ms. Sontag explains the current myth about cancer which proposes that one is responsible for one's disease. This myth applied to tuberculosis as well, before that disease was curable. ". . . the hypothesis that distress can affect immunological responsiveness (and, in some circumstances, lower immunity to disease) is hardly the same as—or constitutes evidence for—the view that emotions cause diseases. . . . Psychological theories of illness are a powerful means of placing the blame on the ill. . . ." There are few of us who have not experienced depression and traumatic events in our lives. I believe that painful feelings are a fact of the human condition and not a necessary prerequisite to cancer.

There was a myth Doren had always had about herself, one which the family had upheld, that she was delicate, too vulnerable. This myth was not realized in her cancer. As hopeless as Doren had felt at various times in her life, she could never give up. When Doren felt beaten down, comfort was drained out of her world. She experienced emotions completely, never holding back on either joy or pain. Doren never relinquished the struggle between vulnerability and strength. When the cancer came and her life was in jeopardy, Doren's warrior spirit never was. Joy was never obliterated by pain, her fight was never relinquished. Doren's optimism shone.

Losing my child was the worst reality I have ever had to face. . . . But the miracle is that I am alive and about to begin again. I have a wonderful new job. It begins on Tuesday.

But most important is that most of the time—although I do feel terribly wounded—I feel like ME again. Me as a strong, capable, desirable creature whose life is not really over.

My commitment to myself feels more solid this time; I pray that I find the strength to follow through on the good things that are before me. I pray that I will be able to see my child soon, and that the next time there *will* be a happy father . . . who is my love.

December 1978. It is late morning and I am in the
shower when the phone rings. I know it is my mother
from the hospital. With news. Benign or malignant. It
is supposed to be benign. I am not supposed to be
worried. Doren is fine. This is just routine surgery to
remove a benign tumor. I jump out of the shower,
leave the water running, do not even grab a towel
although it is a cold December day. I lurch for the
telephone. I don't even say hello. I hear my mother
crying on the other end. I gasp. She murmurs, "It's
cancer." "I'll be right there," I say. I don't remember
hanging up the phone. I scream louder than I have
ever heard myself scream. I fall, naked and soaking
wet, to the floor. Screaming, screaming, screaming.
Neighbors are pounding on my door, asking if I am all
right. I don't remember anything after that until I am
in the hospital room, sitting next to Doren on the bed,
holding her soft hand; she is shaking her head slowly
from side to side, looking into my eyes, tears falling down her face. It is so utterly and impossibly
silent.

April 1980. Doren is well now. Another crazed phone
call from her, complete with more substantial threats,
judgments, innuendo. She is furious that I have been
out of contact with her, because I am choosing
distance in a twenty-eight-year-old relationship.
She thinks I have betrayed her, that I am no longer
her friend, that I have taken a vacation. "I don't
need friends who take vacations from the relationship." She says she is excommunicating me from her
soul. She is trying to control the distance, control
me, with her hostility and anger. I do not have confidence she will ever understand my need to separate from the symbiotic part of our connection.
Distance does not mean severing. It simply means
distance.

I started to run. Six miles every day. I felt I was driving toxins out of my body. I didn't dare miss a day. Running became an obsession. I became a vegetarian. I had devised my own little fairy tale: If I kept this up, I would evade illness. While Doren was in the hospital I would sometimes visit her in the morning after I had finished my run, still in my sweat clothes, drenched and red in the face. She was lying in a hospital bed, wearing a pale hospital gown, with a plastic identification bracelet wrapped around her wrist. The sight of me, blood vehemently coursing through my body, brought her great pleasure.

A doctor said to Doren, "If you were going to get cancer, you got the best kind you can get." He meant that she had a very small tumor, the cancer was isolated, there was no lymph-node involvement, no other involvement at all. The medical lingo entered our lives: Doren was "clean." After culling all the medical opinions, Doren decided on a lumpectomy. A mastectomy was too radical for the kind of tumor Doren had. After the lumpectomy, there would be an iridium implantation—radioactive matter implanted in Doren's breast for a few days, and then removed. During the implantation days, no one was allowed to come near Doren. At least not too near. She and Rob wrote little notes back and forth to each other, and they also drew pictures.

Chickens, sunsets, love in the setting sun, talking till 4:00 in the morning, and then talking some more. These are in his pictures and in her heart. . . .

OOOM-MAH . . . wet kisses from radioactive D.

The sun, the sun, will send its blessing to all of us who have passed the fearful times and still have hope. . . .

Doren and Rob were no longer living together. He returned to his loft, where his former lover still lived. She wouldn't leave. She was co-owner of the loft. Doren hated the situation. She didn't understand why Rob would not extricate himself from a woman he claimed he no longer loved. The bone of contention between Doren and Rob was always this "other woman."

When Doren first became ill and was in the hospital going through the lumpectomy "procedures," Rob was there. When she returned home his presence was inconsistent. Did he feel that Doren was out of danger and that business as usual was the appropriate response? Did I? Surely I must have, given that shortly thereafter I instigated a separation from Doren.

It was after Doren's breast cancer that her journal stopped. Her date book became an abbreviated diary.

WEDNESDAY, DEC. 20. 9:00 A.M. Surgery: Malignant Tumor.

THURSDAY, DEC. 21. 11:30 A.M. Bone Scan.

FRIDAY, DEC. 22. 12 noon. Surgery: Good news. No node involvement. No mirror image.

SATURDAY, DEC. 23/XMAS. Home from hospital. Xmas Eve not too jolly.

MONDAY, DEC. 25. Rob leaves again. Cathy sleeps over.

WEDNESDAY, DEC. 27. Mother sleeps over.

TUESDAY, FEB. 13, 1979. Iridium Implant Procedure. Surgery 2:15. Very hard. Severe nausea.

MONDAY, FEB. 19. SNOW. Out of hospital. Quiet day at home. Feeling much better.

TUESDAY, MARCH 6. Very full day. Feeling better, but night is too empty. It hurts.

Doren was working as an assistant editor at a publishing company. In April, four months subsequent to discovering she had cancer, she was fired from her job. No logical reason was given. Doren had been out ill at various times. There was someone in charge who didn't like this very much, who didn't seem to like the fact that Doren had cancer.

By this time I was not in communication with my sister. Her cancer had drawn me back to her, and to the family, in a way that threatened me. I felt like I was fighting for my own life.

Doren had become more demanding, more intrusive. The only way I knew to deal with this was to completely extricate myself from the relationship. She had no more cancer. Doren was all right now, the doctors said. What I hadn't realized at all was the degree of anger I must have felt. How dare Doren get cancer! How dare she put that kind of scare into my life! I took my energies away from Doren and put them into Jeffrey. Like Rob in Doren's life, Jeffrey was there and not there in my life. Doren and I continued to suffer from the unavailable man syndrome.

I had virtually cut myself off from my family. Just at the point at which I had begun to renew a relationship with my father, I cut myself off from him too. Doren and my father were in close contact. To be in contact with my father would bring me too close to Doren. This was also true with my mother. And I wanted out. I was blaming them for my pain. I needed to be near Jeffrey as much as I felt I needed to get away from my family. My attempts at connection weren't working. I was keeping myself solitary. But even in isolation, I didn't feel safe. I thought, in fact, that Jeffrey was correct in keeping his distance from me. I felt I had no business wanting love. There was no love I was feeling for myself.

April morning. Raining. Chilled. Cotton bathrobe and clogs. No running because of rain.

Don't get too secure, Cathy. Disaster will surely strike. I don't trust. I wonder if I ever will. Will silence and distance always hold the threat of being permanently cut off? The insecurity, the lack of self-confidence, the sound of the Greek chorus runs so deep. At least the leaves are finally coming through on the trees outside my window. I've been watching them. I've been watching something come to life.

After Jeffrey entered my life and Doren became ill, when I wrote about my fear, about distance, about separation, I thought I was referring to Jeffrey. Now I discover that by plucking Jeffrey's name out of a sentence, replacing it with Doren's name, the true feeling comes to light. In so many ways, Jeffrey became the conduit for all of my unexpressed emotions toward my sister.

Rage . . . Had a fantasy last night of buzzing Jeffrey's bell, tromping up the stairs, striding into his apartment and completely tearing it apart. Tapes and tape deck first.

Then phone pulled out of wall and thrown. Then books thrown off shelves, papers and anything else on desks thrown off. Then I imagined myself with a gun. The gun went off. Pop. Small flames came out. I didn't picture Jeffrey falling to the floor or dying. Just that pop.

Absolutes—what I was telling Doren tonight, at our first meeting in months—do not exist in human emotions, in relationships. She thinks they do exist and should exist. Because I have disappointed her, because I am not like her, because I cannot fulfill her needs the way she wants me to, she has condemned and judged me. She thinks she is a better person than I. She says she would never "do to me" what I "did to her." That if I were seriously ill, she'd put all her feelings aside. That her way is the right way, the truly good-person way. BULLSHIT! Jeffrey, you're fucking selfish! Doren, you are too! Both of you are capable of just what I am capable of.

Doren reprimanded me during a dinner we had together at a Japanese restaurant in her neighborhood. It had been six months since the discovery of her breast cancer, and the lumpectomy. The cancer had not returned. Doren's voice was stern, she was unyielding in her judgment of me. I slowly dipped raw fish in hot mustard, my mouth burning as Doren glared at me across the table. Her list of resentments took the form of a litany. It included two periods of our relationship, two periods that she was holding against me. She began with the most recent—my silence subsequent to her lumpectomy. "Did you really think that was it? Did you really think I was fine after that? Don't you think the fact that I have had cancer is affecting me? I can't forgive you for not being there for me all these months."

I explained the only reasons I knew about, at the time, for the separation. I told Doren my identity was so wrapped up with hers. I said nothing about my fear and anger about possibly losing her. She wasn't listening. And I wasn't listening either. We kept a staunch hold on what we believed to be the truth.

Then Doren went even further back. She talked about the first year of her marriage, my first year of college, the way she rallied for me at the expense of her own life—she gave me keys to her apartment, she helped me with schoolwork, she cooked me meals, she talked to me hours on end, she diverted me from fearful thoughts, she made her husband accept a mar-

riage that included her hysterical younger sister. Doren reminded me of all this as I gulped ice water to soothe my
flaming mustard tongue. "So this is what I get in return for
helping you survive that year in Boston," she said. I replied
simply, "I will never be able to give you what you want. If you
were in a hospital and dying, I still couldn't be there for you in
the way you seem to want me to be—I can't sacrifice everything in my life for you."

Little did either of us know the days that were to come.

It was during this time of silence with my family, and Jeffrey's intermittent silence with me, that I returned to acting. I
had begun work on a new novel that I was unable to continue
after Doren's cancer. The novel was autobiographical. There
was no specific reason I remember being aware of that inspired
me to enroll in an acting class. I just knew that someday I had
to return to it, to see how I felt about it now that I no longer
felt the family pressure on me to be an actress. Taking the class
was an experiment I did not want to get too serious about. I
didn't want anything to threaten my identity as a writer. My
teacher, Word Baker, the man who would become one of the
few crucial mentors in my life, saw that I would, one day, have
to take my acting as seriously as my writing. He didn't tell me
this, however. He waited until I discovered it for myself. It
wasn't until later that I found the courage, the necessity, to
accept the two aspects of myself I had always kept apart.

On my twenty-eighth birthday I was at home alone, writing
journal through midnight, looking up occasionally at the photographs on my bulletin board. Doren was now safe, I thought.
I saw myself at five years old, standing fragile and unhappy in
a bathtub, my father having come in to snap my picture; at
nine, beaming, walking down a dirt path at camp on visiting
day between my mother and sister; in my early twenties,
standing on a mountain with a knapsack on my back, celebratory, posing for Doren's ex-husband.

I was trying to reconcile all the aspects of the past in order to
come full into the present. I knew I was in there somewhere,
consistent, but I couldn't yet find that part of myself I could
depend on. It was time, I knew, to begin depending on myself
for stability. That was hard to do, since I had always looked
toward the triumvirate—the merging of my mother, my sister,
and me—for my stability and my focus. The triumvirate was
not foolproof and I had to begin to relinquish my dependency
on it.

Doren's friend, Candice, returned from her archaeological

work in Greece. She had moved back to her parents' farm in Virginia and had brought with her Scott, the man who was now her husband. They had met on one of Candice's many digs. Candice and Scott were living in a small house close to the main house where Candice's mother and father still lived. Then Candice's father died suddenly of a heart attack. There is a notation in Doren's date book on that day. It was made, Doren added later, before she had heard of his death. She felt, therefore, that there was a psychic connection.

<u>Horrible</u>   Horrible   <u>Horrible</u>

Loss

Loss

Loss Loss Loss

Loss Loss Loss

Candice had called Doren the day after her father died. Doren had just been in Virginia the preceding weekend. She was so glad she had seen Candice's father that one last time. The ashes would be buried on the farm, right beside the beautiful vegetable and flower gardens. It would be only two years later that Doren's ashes would be buried on the same land.

Dear Candice—

I am with you in spirit; please let me help you in any way I can. Don't forget about calling *collect* at any hour you need to . . . and let me know when a visit would be appropriate.

I'm so grateful we had our wonderful visit. I'll cherish its warmth always.

Love, Doren

(P.S. to Scott: Thank you for the delicious sandwiches for the train. You are a man in a million.)

I noticed my father was frequently on my mind so I decided it was time to see him. I explained my rule—if he insisted on making my relationship with Doren an issue in my relationship with him, then I would not be able to see him during this time. My father had continued to feel obligated to speak in Doren's behalf, and I couldn't tolerate this. I wanted the other members of my family to trust that I had good reasons for the separation. My father didn't trust me at all, he felt I was being blatantly cruel, and I requested that he simply remain mute on the subject. That first visit veered into a surprising area. My father proceeded, in response to a few of my questions, to explain his version of the family history. The history being his marriage to my mother and the subsequent breakdown and breakup of that relationship. I listened with rapt attention, then rushed home to set it down on paper. Never had I heard it all from my father's point of view. What I had heard from my father, for as long as I could remember, was that he felt I had arrived in the world chock-full of "prenatal hostility." He felt my mother and I were in cahoots way back when her blood was my blood and my fingernails were not even formed yet. My father had not been able to get close to me, and he claimed that when I was a mere infant, I had pushed him away.

The real stress in the marriage began while my mother was pregnant with me. In some ways I became a symbol of that stress. During my meeting with my father I explained to him that I had always felt responsible for the demise of a happy family. This shocked him. He was adamant that I had nothing to do with his problems or the problems in the marriage. He was letting me off the hook.

I knew the truth was somewhere nestled in between my mother's vision, my father's vision, and my sister's vision, not to mention my own, but finally I felt like I had all the pieces— no matter that they were in disarray—in my possession. There was relief in this. I was also proud of myself that I had, for the first time, allowed my father a voice.

During the summer of 1979 I had made up my mind that I was going to run the New York Marathon that October. I began to train. Training, for me, meant pure obsession. Muscles and tendons began to ache, my ankle especially. One doctor told me I had to stop running for two weeks. When I returned home after that appointment I became hysterical. The idea of not running for two weeks was devastating to me, though I didn't understand why this was so. Every day during those two weeks I took my bicycle out—a clunky, three-speed English racer—wrapped the chain that weighed a ton around the seat, and raced around Central Park God knows how many times before seven in the morning. I went to a gym and worked out. I continued to bike all around the city whenever I had to go anywhere. After a steady week of frenzied and excessive exercise, I collapsed. Literally. I couldn't move for the entire month of August. I had severely injured my back and was in agony. I kept pleading for something strong enough to kill the pain. Nothing the doctor prescribed worked. Had morphine been offered me, I don't doubt I would have taken it.

I stayed in my own house during those weeks, refusing to go to my mother's house to be taken care of. That idea seemed much too dangerous; I feared the childlike state I would probably regress to if I was put into my old bedroom and catered to by my mother. My friends came and went, taking shifts, helping me out. Even in the state I was in I managed to arrange and schedule and coordinate to make sure my needs were met. I was that determined not to be brought in such a weakened condition to my mother's home. It was fine with me, however, for her to visit, bring me food, offer support. As long as I was under my own roof, I felt safe.

I felt safe, however, only up to a point. I had never before been betrayed by my body and been rendered physically helpless. It was the first hint of my own mortality, and it shook me up. As I began to heal, I called Doren. I wanted to see her now. This woman who was my sister had had cancer. I finally realized her mortality as well. I would have to work out the things that troubled me about our relationship. I knew I wanted her in my life.

Doren and I were happy about our reconciliation. We were getting along. And then something strange began to happen. Doren became more intrusive than she had ever been. She seemed irrational. Her behavior was so extreme, I could make no sense of it. We had long ago agreed to keep our professional lives separate. Suddenly she was threatening to submit some of her writing to someone who had long been generating work for me. I was outraged. I insisted Doren not make this move. She then tried to contact my therapist, Betty, presumably to talk about me. As it was, Doren had started therapy also, just previous to getting cancer. Her therapist was a close friend of Betty's whom Betty had recommended to Doren. Added to which, my mother was recently in therapy, since Doren's illness, with a woman who knew the two other therapists. In other words, there were three women who knew each other, treating three women who were symbiotic. Two triumvirates. It felt as if everyone knew about everyone else. I was never comfortable with the arrangement. I managed to intercede so that Doren never had the talk with my therapist that she had desired. Then, in very harsh and very angry words, I told Doren to take a walk. I told her I was through with her.

Within days I received a call from my mother.

Doren was very ill.

The cancer had returned.

The notation in Doren's date book is huge, bold, scrawled across the page.

————

THURSDAY, AUG. 30, 1979

B L A C K   D A Y

CANCER HAS SPREAD

————

Doren has cancer. It was detected in her shoulder, lung, brain, and liver. I received the call about the cancerous liver when I was in Betty's office. I had instructed my mother to call me there when she knew of the test results. Choking with fear, sadness, guilt, I was curled like a fetus as Betty held me. This news came at the end of August, beginning of September. I don't know the exact date, nor do I care to know. It is now November. I have stopped choking. Outwardly. I suspect the choking has taken other forms. Doren's doctor feels that, at this point, the chemotherapy and radiation have arrested the cancer. Doren's negative symptoms—infections, fatigue, no appetite, nausea— are *supposedly* (my faith is not at its peak) caused by the treatments. Doren's hair has fallen out. I have not yet seen her bald head. She wears silk scarves and has a red wig she wore only once and hated. She has been accepting, she has raged, she has been accepting again. I can easier talk about her "stages" than my own. Mine are so unclear. When I think about these things, life is so foreign to me. . . .

PRAYER

Let's talk about prayer
doesn't it have phases too?
And how many? Does it fly
out over the small bed   or is it sediment
that stains the inside   of the wine barrel
before the grapes get there?

Some say it could be hair
settling down over the bare skull
of a living woman

my brave hand on your shoulder
has forgotten stunning things

C. S. Lewis writes, "Tonight all the hells of young grief have opened again; the mad words, the bitter resentment, the fluttering in the stomach, the nightmare unreality, the wallowed-in tears. For in grief nothing 'stays put'. One keeps on emerging from a phase, but it always recurs. . . . Everything repeats. Am I going in circles, or dare I hope I am on a spiral? But if a spiral, am I going up or down it? How often—will it be for always?—how often will the vast emptiness astonish me like a complete novelty and make me say, 'I never realized my loss till this moment'?"

I sit here writing with four years of grief behind me and also spread out around me. My desk is covered with it. My journal pages, my poems, Doren's letters, journals, poems, her novel. When I think of Doren I cannot help but think of myself as well. I cannot see the last years of her life clearly. They are so connected to my grief.

I have to keep reminding myself that the years of acute pain have passed. Then they catapult toward me again, threatening to take over and fill me with anguish that has a dreaded familiarity.

Whatever anger I had been seething with before, toward my sister, whatever decision I had made concerning our relationship, was cast into oblivion. All that mattered was Doren's life.

There was more for us to attend to than personal turmoil and the grief that had already begun within my family even though Doren was still alive. There were so many details, so much information that had to be acquired and compiled. Health care, insurance, medical consultations. I had a new file in my drawer labeled: CANCER CARE. I had taken the responsibility of finding out what services were available for Doren at home. She was intent on staying at her apartment. I took notes on every phone call. I made a record of every conversation, wrote down the names of everyone I spoke to, the date I spoke to them. There were various social service departments at various hospitals, records were being transferred, homemaker services were being contacted, home nursing care was lined up. One notation reads: "9/5—Spoke to Mrs. Goldman. If we need someone this weekend, we must let her know tonight. Her home phone is . . . If a nurse is needed for a period of 24 consecutive hours, she only gets paid for 12 hours—that is, if the patient is not in need of her assistance for the other 12 hours when, presumably, the nurse can sleep. If Doren needs actual (active) assistance over 24 hours—meaning the nurse must assist her through the night—another nurse comes in to take the second shift. And so, we must make clear our needs. Price: $35/day (sleep-in, one nurse), during the week (Sun. night–Fri. night); $40/day (sleep-in, one nurse) on the weekend."

The details were serving the purpose of keeping me from myself, and that was just the thing I wanted to be kept from. My family was doing the same. We all had our various chores around illness to keep us preoccupied. We became obsessive about those chores, and when we would get together for discussions we talked in furious circles, pretending we were figuring everything out, pretending we were controlling death.

Doren was still Doren. Having cancer did not suddenly transform her into a person whose essential identity was "cancer victim." Some people who have never experienced a crisis of this enormity wonder how it is possible to get through it. I discovered that you just simply continue being you. Doren was still Doren, she just happened not to be feeling well. She continued to live in the most productive way she could under the circumstances. Her life came first, the circumstances of her illness came second. I suspect that we, those who were around her, followed her example. No matter how much pain, no matter the moments of overwhelming fear, life did continue.

I was hesitant about keeping a journal during this time. I was sure that writing down my feelings would exacerbate the pain. Betty reminded me—if you filter your emotions through your creative process, you will be reunited with your own power.

I was in the danger zone this past weekend. Doren going into the hospital for blood transfusions on Wednesday; me just avoiding getting mugged on Thursday night; seeing a woman lying on the road in Central Park on Sunday. A time when the danger button is too close at hand, when the next image or thought could push it, when I could be sucked into the dark side of all things. . . .

Mother just called to ask if I wanted to join her and George for dinner. Once again, as on Sunday, I start to cry when we acknowledge our fears about Doren. I am still crying. It feels like it is about Doren. About feeling so alone. About *being* alone . . .

Another call from Mother. She has spoken to Doren's doctor. He continues to have good news to report about the cancer in her lungs clearing. He says he is encouraged. Am I afraid to be hopeful?

On March 22, 1982, exactly one year after Doren died, I remembered something that had occurred between us during this time immediately following the second cancer diagnosis. I lit a candle and sat at my typewriter. It was the typewriter that had belonged to my sister. I lit a candle and took out the picture of Doren that I always kept hidden between the pages of my appointment book. I needed to talk to her.

Doren, I remember that day with you in the bagel restaurant—we were on our way to the doctor's office. We had just come from the hospital where you had bone scans. You didn't yet know that your doctor was going to tell you that you would need not only chemotherapy but brain radiation as well. And it was all going to begin happening to you within twenty-four hours. Within a matter of days your hair would start falling out. I already had all this information, and my task was to get you to a store that day, before going to the doctor's office, to get you a wig. You didn't want to do that. You didn't know what the rush was. You had started chemotherapy and had been told it would be a while before your hair fell out. You felt weak. I walked a block with you very slowly, helping you cross a street, watching you to make sure you were all right. And then you said you wanted to eat. That's when we found the bagel place. But I thought getting that wig was so crucial. I gave in, finally, to what you really wanted to do. Fuck the wig, I thought. And you got a huge bagel sandwich. And it made you so incredibly happy. I didn't eat anything. I watched you. There were times that last year when I watched you so hard. Studied you. I wanted to memorize you. Especially your hands. In the last months, the last weeks, I memorized your hands, looking at them, touching them, massaging them. I just knew I didn't want to forget those hands. That day, watching you eat your bagel sandwich, I saw a glow radiating from your face. You caught my eye. We looked at each other. There was an overwhelming euphoria between us. "Doren," I said, "I just want you to know that I know. I know." You were so happy, you said, "How do you know what I'm thinking?" "I just do." "I know you do," you said. We didn't dare put words to the feeling. It was impossible. We were talking about the connection of our spirits, the connection that was eternal. In that moment of awareness there was no death. There was excitement. We knew we would always be together. That in whatever way spirits were connected, ours were. The awareness and acknowledgment of that kinship was so comforting, our love for each other immense and deep.

1962. I am fifteen. An early February morning in Merrick: I have the feeling, and it gets stronger with time, that there is somewhere a truth, a way of looking at things that will change the whole perspective of history and man himself. But I also feel that, although poets and artists may search for it, no one has yet done more than touch it briefly. It has not yet been realized fully by the living but I just know (I don't know where I got this idea) that when a person dies he knows forever. That sounds crazy, and it's difficult to express, but I think it's the essence of my religion and philosophy. When I say I want to be the greatest writer (what ambition) I mean that I want to achieve the outlook and fulfill it before I die. I *must*—at least I must die trying.

Relatives came to New York from out of town during the first couple of weeks of September 1979. Given the diagnosis, everyone thought Doren might go at any minute. Everyone around her looked wan, dazed. Doren, on the other hand, looked beautiful, robust as ever, gleaming. It was surely impossible that Doren was dying. My God, she didn't look ill at all.

Doren requested that pictures be taken of her. This was the day in the Village, posing, watching my sister pose. Rob was there too. Rob and Doren posed together while I snapped their picture. I was shivering. It was late afternoon. I was dressed for summer, wearing a thin pink jacket. Doren was dressed in a cashmere sweater and a warm skirt. She was sensible. She had planned ahead.

My aunt had brought beautiful antique jewelry for Doren. Some of it my aunt had always worn, some had long been in a drawer. Sibling rivalry did not evade me. I felt jealous and was in shock that I did. In time I learned that such an inclination would never pass from my body, even when Doren was gone. I do not stop being Doren's sister, even in this way.

We were not always bleak. We still had fun like we always had, and we did not evade humor. Doren, Mother, George, and I were all watching television one night. Suddenly I turned to Doren and blurted out, "Leave it to you to even get cancer first!" There was a moment when everyone looked startled, and then there was laughter. As we were all still laughing, I continued, "Now if *I* get it, it'll be no big deal! No one will pay attention to me at all!"

Toward the end, when it became increasingly difficult for Doren to walk from one room to another while she was staying at my mother's apartment, I'd often help her to the bathroom. When she was ready for me to come and bring her back to her bed, she'd buzz a buzzer that had long been an unused fixture in the apartment, from a time, decades earlier, when presumably there had been servants. She'd turn to me when I appeared and, with a blasé flick of her wrist in the air, she'd say coolly, "Flush, peon."

I remember her in the blue nightshirt she had taken home from the Medical Center, and in her red Chinese slippers, padding into my mother's kitchen through the swinging pantry door. She had become so thin, and she was bending over because it hurt to stand straight. Doren looked up at us sitting at the table and smiled mischievously. "Look at this," she said, and she began to swivel her hips and shuffle her feet back and forth in place. "It's called the Medical Center shuffle."

Just after Doren began her chemotherapy and radiation treatments, she received her first book contract. The book she was planning to write would be called *Good Girls;* it would be a rewrite of the earlier novel she had written, and shelved, while she was married to Andrew. Feelings of jealousy rose up. Doren's book will be going out into the world before one of mine, I thought. I will, as always, have to follow her act, live up to her talent, withstand the comparisons, always feel that I am second in command. How can I feel this way? I berated myself. My sister is probably dying of cancer and I am envious of her success. For a while I felt so ashamed.

My guilt abated somewhat. I managed to stop blaming Doren for getting a contract for a book before me. If you're so goddamn competitive, I said to myself, why don't you just finish writing your own? Perhaps competition is not so sinful, I thought.

Doren arranged a party to celebrate the signing of her book contract. This was at the start of her chemotherapy and radiation treatments and they were making her violently ill. She wasn't feeling well at all the night of the party but she was determined to be a gracious hostess. That night was the only time she wore the red wig. It occurred to me that it looked like my hair. I asked Doren if there was any chance she was trying to look like me. She started to laugh. "You could be right on that," she admitted. This was the first time I had ever caught a glimpse of Doren's competition with me. I found it hard to understand. I had always felt she was the beautiful one. Later she would tell me the reverse was true for her.

To utilize my competitive spirit in an area that was separate from my sister, I kept to my plan to run the marathon. The night before the event, my mother and George were married. They had been living together for years. I knew that part of the reason they were marrying at this time was that my mother wanted Doren to be there for this happy event in her life. It was a modest ceremony at their apartment, with family and close friends. I took dozens of pictures. After Doren died, when I would look at them, I would be hit with the marked change in my mother's appearance. She looks so beautiful and joyous and clear in those pictures. Her smile takes over her face. I wondered whether she'd ever look that way again. Doren is in only one photograph. She is wearing a pink and red silk scarf and sunglasses. The light hurt her eyes. There is no smile.

With barely any training (except for one long run two weeks before the race), my bad back (which I feared would give out at any minute), and absolutely no sleep the night before, I joined what amounted to a moving city on an extremely hot October day. I wasn't exactly in my right mind. I sat among thousands in a large park on Staten Island waiting for the race to begin. I had brought paper and pen with me.

> New York City Marathon. 21 October 1979. A night of no sleep. My knees are weak. My face is flushed. Ate half a plain doughnut and felt ill. . . . The man next to me is concentrating on *The New York Times* Sunday crossword puzzle. This is all surreal. Fourteen thousand people. Challenge. My own. Testing my will, which must set up residence in my body. Connected. Nothing within me must be alienated from anything else within me. Jeffrey says I am not stopping the world today. I am stopping *my* world. Holding it. Doing something else with it. The world inside. Taking hold.

Before the race I thought: If at any point I feel I can't go on, all I have to do is think about Doren. Her will is keeping her alive. I'm calling upon my own to do a lot less than that. Doren was too ill to come out and watch me run. I was dedicating my own personal marathon to her.

Whoever comes into contact with Doren usually ends up exclaiming to her how courageous she is. One day Doren says to me, "I don't understand why they say this. What do they expect? What else am I to do? Here are my choices: Either I give up, or I live. I am only choosing to live. I don't see what that has to do with courage." We are crossing a street in the Village, returning to Doren's apartment after having dinner at her favorite Japanese restaurant. Doren turns to me and whispers, "Don't tell anyone, but I've never felt so wonderful about myself as I do now. I've never been happier. That sounds crazy, but do you understand?"

There is sorrow somewhere above sea level. We have acknowledged this, on our way to the mountains. If we forget, the storm, shaped like a large, nameless animal, passing over the mountain range, will remind us. When it grazes the border of a white cumulus cloud, we will feel the necessary shifting. So we know this even when we follow the movement of gold light that looks like a star, that might embody small amounts of time, like hours, as we do, because it is staying with us. We keep seeing it. It must be moving with us, disappearing, appearing again, higher this time, but there, still there, and what we don't dare admit yet is that we must also, in those gaping moments, be lost to the light we feel is lost to us.

A leopard could suddenly appear on the road, leaping out of possible danger into a rising ice-jungle. And the weather station on top of Mt. Washington is secured to the ground with chains.

I spent the winter of 1979 virtually alone and in movie theaters. My calendar was marked with double features every day in every "revival" movie theater in New York. I was seeing every old movie I had never seen. I was now a free-lance story analyst for New York offices of film studios and major networks and was fitting in a lot of work between Charlie Chaplin and Mae West. I was also singing. I had signed up for a singing class, as well as an acting class, at Herbert Berghof Studio. During the week I would rehearse with a pianist, and on the weekend, in class, I'd sing Rodgers and Hart, and Cole Porter.

Candice—

Happy 1980!
Thank you so much for the splendid gifts—all delightful and useful (Rob was very moved by his incredibly original gift of a horseshoe; he put it over his front door). I'm feeling wonderful (no medicine for 3 weeks) and wishing you and Scott would come to N.Y.C. for a few days. . . . Saw your friends in Westchester and bought some lovely pottery. . . . How's tricks?

love, Doren

This is where I want to be tonight. New Year's Eve. At my desk. My typewriter. Surrounded by my writing, my poetry, my novels, and the poetry of Robert Bly, W. S. Merwin. My spiritual guides. I didn't speak to Doren today. Feel bad about that now. I love my sister. I want her to be well. I don't want her to die. She has a right to live out her life, to become well again. I pray for her. I pray to whatever spirit there is in this world, and I know there is spirit, there must be a vortex where all spirit joins—I pray to that place, that strength, to nurture Doren, to nourish her in all ways that are necessary to help make her well.

It was a cold, brutal winter, always dark it seemed. Doren was getting injections, taking pills, having transfusions, losing weight. I was annoyed with her that she enjoyed being skinny. I wanted her to eat more. I wanted to see her fill out again. I cried often without realizing the source of my sadness was grief. I thought it was about Jeffrey, who I was no longer seeing.

24 January 1980. I can't stand it. Earlier I felt: How do I live my life without him? I swear I don't know how. I swear I don't want to.

It doesn't stop, this love.

All those people wearing kerchiefs in my dreams in the last two weeks. The image becomes clear when I start telling Doren and I am staring right at her head, covered with a hat. Turbans. Scarves. Kerchiefs. The silken strips of cloth threatening to go into orbit without me. Doren is in all these dreams.

27 January 1980. I marvel at Doren's positiveness and wonder how I would cope with a similar hardship. I'm so tied in with my physical energy, with trying to be in control over my body. My back accident was certainly traumatic for me, and although I hope that I would, next time, cope more positively with a physical malady, I really don't know. I seem to be relying on running again.

Missing Jeffrey is cutting me too deep and yet he remains with me no matter what I do.

Doren was having a great deal of difficulty concentrating on writing. Her days were so unpredictable. She would feel all right and strong one hour and be vomiting the next. The illness was isolating her enough without the additional isolation a writer must bear. Doren went to see a film one day called *Best Boy*. It was a poignant story about a man who was retarded. Doren was seized with an idea. The story was a true one and she visited the school for retarded adults that the man in the film had attended. She volunteered her services to teach.

She did not tell the people she worked for, or with, about the cancer. No one questioned why she always wore a scarf. Doren was substitute teaching three or four times a week. If at any point during the day she felt ill, she'd simply excuse herself discreetly and go to the ladies' room. Then she'd return to her "trainees" and continue.

Doren called me frequently with stories of her day, the attachments she was forming with her trainees. She was overjoyed—never had she felt so fulfilled. Her descriptions were vivid, loving. I didn't know how Doren could withstand the sadness of the profound retardation of the adults she was teaching. But if there was sadness, Doren had risen above it. Her trainees were extraordinary and wonderful people, and she was helping them to rise above their own limitations.

Doren had mentioned, only once and briefly at that, the fear about not being able to have children if she survived the cancer. The drugs were killing her chances ever to become pregnant. I don't think this was something she actually accepted as fact, but she had found another route for mothering. She had discovered long ago, as a teenager, how satisfying it was for her to teach special people, and now she had found her way back. These people became the most crucial part of Doren's life before she died. They were her children. She did not complete *Good Girls*—the teaching became her truest life source.

There were visits to Candice on the farm over weekends when she felt well enough, and Rob was still Doren's companion. The relationship no longer troubled Doren in the way it had before. She was no longer relying on it for sustenance.

My sister was not choosing a relationship with death. She was coming full into herself and her life with exuberance. The bouts of illness between chemotherapy treatments were merely a nuisance to her.

7/3
Dear Candice—

Yes, I was a bit tuckered out after our weekend, but I was also so happy to have been with you. It made me realize how much I've missed you over the years; visits (both ways) must be more frequent from now on. Love to Scott, and the horses, Wellworth, Maggie, Pixie, Pirate & Co. Maybe I can visit again in late August. I miss you, friend.

love, Doren

8/5
Dear Candice—

God, it's hot here too! The week when it was past 100° almost every day was an Edgar Allan Poe nightmare to me. Rob kept saying "This is great! Doesn't bother me a bit!" Still, he didn't seem to mind taking refuge in my air-conditioned pied-à-terre. . . .

Rob and I saw the Picasso show a few weeks ago. It's quite an experience, to put it mildly. I frankly have never been a real devotee, but my esteem and sense of wonder at his prodigiousness now is boundless. The portraits, the stone sculpture, the range of styles, even the latest works (early 1970s) are so *fine,* so strong. It's as if he were ten or twelve unique artists living inside one skin. . . .

My doctor continues to be pleased with my response to the medicine. Generally, I feel pretty good, with a few really low-energy days in every month. Pretty soon I will be going on a new "maintenance" regime which, if I am lucky, will allow my hair to grow back again. You can't imagine how I look forward to that. . . .

My book is driving me crazy, but I keep trying to write something interesting. Some days it seems okay, some days like the worst garbage. I have decided to stop throwing out as much as I have been in the hope that I am being too harsh a critic. . . .

Do you think we might come for a visit sometime in September?

Love to Scott—Love to you—Doren

Rob—Va Va Voom! What a night! XO, Baldie

MARILYN HAD THE RIGHT IDEA

Thank God for air conditioners. Without
mine I'd be in Bellevue. Last night
I asked my boyfriend if he thought
divorced women might be especially
susceptible to heat, and he told me
to turn over.

I suppose the summer is rough for
lots of folks—all us depressives.
Immoderate sun making us take off
our clothes, walk around the city
in near-naked bodies whether or not
those bodies spent the winter being
loved. It hurts. No one ever speaks
of the courage of the fat woman in a
sundress, or of the fat man (with
flesh like squeezed toothpaste)
in his Côte d'Azur bikini.

In *The Seven Year Itch*
Marilyn Monroe tells Tom Ewell
that she keeps her undies in the
fridge when the weather gets torrid.
Clever Marilyn. I'd like to put
my head there days like this.
I'd like to ask the sun
to take a walk.

20 May 1980. Doren went to her usual chemotherapy treatment today after her usual two-week rest period, and the doctor said she could go another two weeks without the drugs. First time he has done this. Aren't you worried? Doren asks him. No, I'm not worried, he says. This news brings substance and meaning into my otherwise unconscious day.

My resolve to stay away from Jeffrey didn't hold. By the summer of 1980 I was trying, once again, to work out our relationship. There was comfort I received from being with him. He was someone who understood my feelings about my sister, her illness, my fear of her dying. There were very few people I could talk to about all of these things, very few people who wanted to hear. He couldn't give me all of what I wanted, but I couldn't yet bear to lose what he *could* give.

Doren was in remission, we were told. By the end of the summer I felt the need to get away, and yet I knew I was inept when it came to exits and sticking to them. It was at that point that California loomed large for me. I saw it as a way OUT. Go to California and stay in California. Just get yourself to California.

My work as a free-lance story analyst in New York had expanded my professional world. I had come into contact with people in the movie and television business in Los Angeles who perhaps could help me find similar work there.

I entered the surreal world of Hollywood sets, sound stages, deserted streets, hills. I lunched in studio commissaries, got lost in gigantic supermarkets, drove the freeways at seventy miles an hour blasting rock 'n' roll, blasting out grief.

After a couple of weeks in L.A., I decided I wanted to stay for at least one month more so that I could decide if this was a place I would want to live permanently in. I found an apartment I could sublet for that period of time and returned to New York briefly to take care of miscellaneous details.

Just days before I was due to return to L.A., disaster struck again. Doren's cancer had returned. The remission was over. There was a tumor on her liver. The family was informed of this, but Doren was not. She was feeling all right, so it seemed pointless, cruel, to give her this information right then.

I talked with Doren and I made her promise that if she needed me either to stay, or to return once I had left, she would let me know. We made a pact. Doren was only encouraging. She wanted me to live my life. She had no intention of holding me back for any reason.

"Go do your life," her doctor told me when I asked for his advice as to what to do. "She knows you too well," he said, "she'll suspect something is very wrong if you suddenly change your plans and stay in New York." This sounded right. No one was accusing me of trying to escape, so why should I accuse myself?

En route to L.A., at the end of November. Tchaikovsky's *Pathétique* in my ears. I don't dare cry about Doren. She showed me her bald head last night. Startling. Though after a few minutes, she looked attractive. It was good to see her forehead again instead of it being covered by a scarf. But from the back, she looked like a martian. I feel she knows about the test results on an unconscious, spiritual, and physical level. I feel I'm receiving signals from her similar to the spiritual exchange we had a year ago. And I know she's afraid right now. It was so difficult leaving my house today. I think my feelings about Doren were a large part of the reason why.

Two weeks after I had returned to L.A., my sister found out the cancer remission was over. She had some sort of horrific attack in the middle of the night and was taken from her apartment in an ambulance—sitting up, I was told by both my parents, because the pain made it impossible for her to lie down. I was left with the image of my sister being carried down six flights of stairs in her building, during the cold night, in a chair. What was I doing three thousand miles away?

Still, various people I had come to trust told me it was okay to stay where I was. The phrase was: "There's nothing you can do, nothing is going to happen right away." I think that was a euphemism for: Death was not going to happen just then. I was actually being told what death was going to or not going to do. I knew this presumption about death was not something that would be wise for me to trust.

But I had no clarity. Doren, too, from her hospital bed, was telling me it wasn't necessary to cut my trip short. She would tell me if she needed me. I called everybody I could think of for advice. I had no idea what to do, and I was searching for the right decision. The focus became: Does Doren need me?

That focus changed one day at sunset, facing the Pacific Ocean. I remember sandpipers. I was wearing a red thermal sweatshirt, boots with zippers up the sides. The sky was pastel pink and powder blue. I wanted to stay put. I wanted things to be different. New York held pain, fear, and loss. I wrote in my journal, sitting on the damp beach, and when I looked up a thick fog had suddenly engulfed me. I got up and had to somehow find my way back to my car in all this whiteness. I thought: I'm going home. I want to see Doren. I want to be with her. I stopped thinking about what it was Doren needed and realized a need that was all my own.

When I entered her hospital room in New York, she looked beautiful to me. I was never so sure of where I wanted to be, never so happy to be in any one place, and I don't think that kind of unabashed, explicit clarity has returned to me since that time.

I despise this apartment I grew up in, that Mother still lives in. I wish she and George had moved when they began living together, or when they married. It has the same darkness it had when I was twelve, when my parents were still together, still at war. The bedroom Doren and I shared is now George's office. But he has barely made it his own. It still looks like our bedroom. And the dining room has the ticky-tacky bookshelves my father installed. And the same old couch. And the black patent-leather easy chair my grandfather made. And now Doren is sleeping on a mattress on the dining room floor. It is more comfortable for her than a bed. She is too ill now to be living alone in her own apartment. Mother is buying baby food and making Jell-O, praying Doren will eat *something*. But she won't. She can't. I sit in the dark room with Doren, keeping her company, watching another rerun of *All In the Family*. The shows Doren always hated to watch are now all she can tolerate. I swear to God I will never watch another sitcom as long as I live. For weeks I've been watching them with Doren. Watching sitcoms, and watching her die.

When I arrive tonight to visit with Doren, she is sitting in Grandfather's patent-leather chair, a pillow propped up behind her, her head lowered, her hand covering her face. She won't speak. I ask her what is wrong. She won't say a word. I find my mother. What happened? I ask. I am told that a friend of Doren's visited. She had not seen Doren in over a month, and when she arrived she could not contain her shock. Doren's friend started screaming, "Oh my God! You've lost so much weight! You look awful! Oh my God!" Doren was rendered speechless. Her friend left quickly. Minutes later, Doren's rage exploded. No one could get near her. She began to throw things. Scream. Curse. Cry. She finally became exhausted.

And so she was sitting in that chair, quietly; angry, sad, shutting down.

*T*here are manuals in bookstores explaining death, breaking it down into discernible, logical stages. There is this stage, they say, and then that stage, which gives way to another stage. I bought these books. I thought I had better be conscientious about death. I wasn't admitting Doren was actually dying. None of us were. But I thought I had better put myself on the right track—I had better arm myself with reason.

These books were maddening. They had been leading me to believe that my sister was dying wrong. She wasn't passing through the stages as they were outlined. She wasn't sitting down with her loved ones and talking reasonably about her death.

I believe one must relinquish the idea of logic, of emotional stages clearly discernible in either the one who is dying or the one who is grieving. Doren's dying, if that's what it was, had nothing to do with anything I read about. It wasn't death I was watching. Her dying was comprised of moments of life.

When I threw the books away I began to listen. To listen to Doren, and to be quiet. Doren did not name death. If it was something I wanted her to name, it was not my right to manipulate her needs in order that mine be served. Only vaguely, once or twice, did Doren allude to her own death. And when she did, she had no desire to pursue the matter into any form of discussion.

One night we sat together in my mother's bedroom. I sat on the edge of the bed, Doren sat in an easy chair. This was just before she entered the hospital for the last time. She was painfully thin, the silk scarf still on her head, her eyes so large. She suddenly mentioned that she and her therapist, that afternoon, had begun to broach the subject of death. I was silent for a moment, then asked, "And what was it you said?" Doren snapped at me, "It's none of your business! I don't want to talk about it."

Time belonged to Doren, it was hers to shape in whatever way she needed to. Sometimes her rage was clear, loud, but it was rarely expressed in relation to her illness. When she became dissatisfied with the behavior of those closest to her, she would voice, loudly, her dissatisfaction. I was once berated for running first and coming to see her second. She was so angry at me I thought she'd never want to see me again. At the beginning I would defend myself. Then I saw the futility in that. I learned to allow Doren her anger, even if her anger made no rational sense to me. Dying has nothing to do with what we perceive as rational.

Doren and I were often together in a silence of her choosing. I would massage her hands, her feet, and in those moments she would become aware of parts of her body that were not in pain. Sometimes she'd be able to fall asleep as my hands pressed gently. Nothing needed to be said between us. There was a knowledge in our bodies. If I remained silent, I felt it move through me. My hands on Doren's body kept me connected to that knowledge. Doren and I were sharing the last moments of her life. It is death that is impossible to share. And so, when Doren was no longer with me, it was death that kept returning to my dreams, it was death I kept trying to take hold of as if somehow a connection to Doren in death would ease my sorrow.

It was Christmas when I returned from L.A. to be with my sister. I hadn't expected to be in New York during the holidays, so I hadn't bought any gifts. I had one day in which to shop. Off I went to Bloomingdale's with my charge card. I tore through various departments, barely aware of what I was purchasing. I was on the main floor when suddenly I looked up and saw a huge bright light shining in my face. Before I could discern what this light was, there was a microphone at my mouth. The woman holding the microphone was asking, "Would you mind answering a few questions for *NBC News?*" I was stunned. I said nothing. A crowd was gathering. "We'd like to know why some people save all their Christmas shopping for the last minute. Could you tell us what *your* reasons are for buying gifts on the day before Christmas?"

Dare I? For a few seconds I thought of what would happen if I told the truth. "Well, you see, I hadn't expected to be in town, but then I found out my sister is dying of cancer, so I had to come back, and now I must buy my family Christmas gifts, and I'm thinking of getting my sister a pair of sparkly purple stockings which I know she'll love but I doubt she'll ever get to wear."

That wasn't, however, what I said. I smiled, I gestured, I went on about how much easier it was to shop the day before Christmas because you didn't have time to be picky and wonder if what you were buying for someone was the right thing . . . everything went that much faster . . . it was so much more efficient than spreading it out over so many weeks. . . . "I *love* to do all my Christmas shopping last minute, in one day!" I beamed. The interviewer was pleased. The crowd was pleased. I was amazed.

I went home and called my family, Doren, too, and any friends I could think of, to watch the evening news. I watched myself on television, amazed at how lucid I was and that I even *looked* good. *That* is a person in crisis, I said to myself. There are other people watching me right now, other people in the country who are suffering tragedies, they are looking at me and they are thinking I am just as happy as can be, not a care in the world, that young woman knows nothing about what it's like to feel awful at Christmas.

After that I could no longer look at everybody I saw around me and imagine they were happy and untouched by tragedy. I couldn't feel singled out. I knew tragedy was not developed especially for me.

Doren had bought her Christmas presents early. They were all wrapped before she entered the hospital in December. No one was left out. She had sent a gift to Candice and Scott in Virginia.

12/20
Candice & Scott—

A capful of this potion will turn your bath into a sensual treat. Plus it smells divine and is bluer than the Mediterranean. Plus— it's a wonderful muscle relaxer. Enjoy your baths, and enjoy your holidays.

Fa la la la la
la la la
la—
Doren

I bought Doren the purple stockings. I also bought her shoes for spring that she had asked for. She loved them. She tried them on. She talked about wearing them in a few months. She also talked about visiting Candice at the farm in the spring and asked if I'd join her. I had never been to the farm and Doren wanted to share her favorite place with me.

I had to return the shoes after Doren died in March. When I went to the farm to bury Doren's ashes, I had no doubt she was there with me.

Doren did not tell even her closest friends how ill she was. My parents and I wondered whether we should inform Candice, her mother, and Scott that Doren's illness was accelerating. We knew they would want to see her.

Doren was not losing hope. She never believed she would die. Neither did we. If it happened, we would have to believe it then. But not before. Even when her doctor told us the worst, we didn't relinquish hope. Relinquishing hope would have meant we were relinquishing Doren.

I was on my best behavior with my friends. I knew that if I let myself go, I would become like white water, raging and out of control, toppling anything that touched me.

There were only a few people I could confide in, only a few who were willing to open themselves up to something so painful. There were other casualties that came with the major casualty. These were the friends I lost, the people who could not tolerate the entrance of illness and death into their lives. My close friend Emily was one of these people. Emily fell out of my life as inexplicably as if she had been scooped away into a fourth dimension. At first she had left daily messages on my phone machine. I would return from the hospital at the end of the day and hear Emily on my tape, singing funny songs, reciting dialogue from humorous plays. Her voice was comfort in the silence of my apartment. After a few weeks I noticed that I wasn't *seeing* Emily. We weren't really talking either, except when she would "check in" and I would be called upon to fill her in on what was happening. I couldn't just launch into news reports, and I didn't want to insult her by not saying anything. I'd make plans to see her, but she was very busy. She began to cancel plans with me or, worse, forget we had even made them. My free time was so precious, so rare, that when a plan on a free evening fell through, and with it my much needed distraction, it was no small disappointment. I finally decided I was no longer willing to fill Emily in on aspects of my life she was apparently unwilling to be a part of. I explained to her, over the phone, that there were a few people I was spending time with and talking to, and that I would call her when I was ready to do that. Then Doren died. I never heard from Emily again. I have always felt our relationship would have had a chance had she admitted her difficulty. I suppose she believes the irreparable rift was my fault. I gave her an out. She grabbed it.

During the last weeks of Doren's life, I had taken on a most unusual free-lance assignment. It involved reading pornographic literature. A well-known writer, who had written sev-

eral books on the sexual fantasies of men and women, hired
me to sift through and chart her mail. My finances were low at
the time, and she was paying me well. I had to read letters
people had written to her describing their sexual fantasies and
their feelings in response to her latest book. My job was to put
all these responses into categories—categories of type, categories of fantasies. Most of the letters were from people who
were very disturbed about the content of their sexual fantasies
and, as far as I could discern, had every reason to be.

I was going to the hospital every day, watching Doren, waiting, still in disbelief, then returning home to piles of dirty
letters. I solicited the help of Jeffrey, with whom I was spending time during those weeks, and my mother and George. We
were all reading dirty letters and it made our lives seem even
more surreal and bizarre. The emotional shifts and leaps I had
to make at that time are more astounding to me now, however,
than they were then. I raged about all the people in these
letters who would never get the help and advice they needed,
and I raged about my sister. I became filled with a deep sense
of inappropriateness if I became titillated by any of the fantasies. And, with Jeffrey, I would surrender into our sexual relationship, allowing those feelings to drown all the others.

When Doren entered the hospital for the last time, it was
presumably to receive a new treatment. A last-ditch effort. It
was only her liver they were treating now. There was no telling
whether or not the cancer had spread to other parts of her body
as well, and additional X rays were unnecessary under the
circumstances. If they couldn't fix her liver, there was no point
in trying to fix anything else.

The tumor on Doren's liver was a large, rock-hard presence.
I felt it once. Doren wanted me to. When I put my hand on the
right side of her stomach, I thought of the horrid cells, and I
thought of Doren's good cells, and I imagined the death cells
disintegrating, leaving her body, the good cells taking over.
Doren had taught me this. She closed her eyes, put her hand
on the cancer, concentrated her will over the will of the disease, imagined her body clear and well. Doren also had relax-
ation tapes her therapist had recorded for her. She listened to
them, imagined herself on a beach, listening to the ocean, or
on a mountain, feeling the wind. Doren was discovering ways
to be calm, withstand pain, dissolve anger she believed was
toxic to her body, to her well-being. Doren was teaching me
during the last year of her life how to let go, how not to embrace the negative parts of myself, how not to panic over that

which was not in my control. She entered into a freer spirit and was leading me into my own.

2 FEBRUARY 1981
Time alone with Doren. I sit on the edge of the tub while she is taking a bath. Now she keeps her scarf off in front of me. We talk about camp, we sing camp songs. She mentions God.

3 FEBRUARY 1981
Doren's doctor talks to us. He says the words: Doren is dying. Mother cries. I cry. We are able to connect instead of staying alone with our grief. It is the first time we cry together.

With Doren tonight. She tells me how much I am helping, how wonderful I've been. I tell her it feels better being with her than not being with her.

5 FEBRUARY 1981
Afternoon news comes of new treatment planned for Doren. Hope is so strong in taking over. Tonight Doren eats well. Faith seems to have returned to her. Hope still does have a place here.

7 FEBRUARY 1981
This afternoon Doren and Rob and I go to the French restaurant on the corner. Incredible that Doren is dressed, wearing makeup, good clothes. I think this is the hope of the new treatment. She smiles; lively moments.

8 FEBRUARY 1981
I sing '60's songs to Doren, plus disco. She sings along with me, and then we are back to singing camp songs.

11 FEBRUARY 1981
Bring Doren to hospital this afternoon. She is in trauma, so disoriented. The room she is in is so depressing. I come home early and try to work. This depth of pain is frightening.

14 FEBRUARY 1981
With Doren, morning. We sing; mostly I sing to her. Her disorientation gets worse. Jeffrey says it's the drugs.

Call tonight from Gene, an old friend of Doren's from Walden. He is in town. He heard from a mutual friend what is happening to Doren. He wants to help.

There are Valentine cards taped to the wall in front of Doren's bed so she can see them. When Doren is given a shot for the pain and the needle, too, is painful, I sing to her and make her sing with me, "Peace I ask of thee, oh river; peace, peace, peace. . . ."

Gene was in New York on business. He offered his support, his warmth, his affection. He met me before and after my visits to the hospital, he took me out for meals, managed to distract me. One night, at midnight, I was seized with the desire to see Doren. Gene took me in a cab to the hospital, he helped to sneak me up to Doren's floor, he waited for me in the hallway (I didn't want him to see Doren—I knew it would hurt him too much), and then he took me home. I wasn't able to sleep. I couldn't stop shaking. Gene stayed with me through the night, stroking my forehead, comforting me into sleep. The next morning we cried together. Gene loved Doren too.

My cat, who had been with me for twenty years, was also dying. She was in and out of the veterinary hospital, getting treatments, being well briefly, and then becoming ill again. I was going back and forth to the hospital to see my sister, and back and forth to the veterinarian with my dying cat. The vet did not suggest I put my cat to sleep, so I watched her waste away. My parents and I were furious at the doctors, who would not increase Doren's painkillers at the end. The doctors were afraid the drugs would kill her. It was insane. She was dying anyway. By refusing to authorize the necessary amount of drugs that would ease her pain, they were condoning her suffering. The confusing and tumultuous feelings I was experiencing regarding my sister's treatment were being projected onto my cat. I wanted them both to be saved. I felt helpless and guilty that they were both in pain.

3 MARCH 1981
Doren is so much a part of me. I feel her gestures in my gestures, her expressions in my expressions, her body in my body, her voice in my voice, her laugh in my laugh, her sadness and happiness mingled with mine. I can't fathom how much I'm going to miss her. Even her voice. Never to hear my sister's voice again. All the moments I'll want to call her, share things with her. Her laugh. I'll miss

her laugh. Her eccentricities. I'll miss them too. There is no one else in the world like Doren.

Rob says tonight she is still the most beautiful woman in the world. He says when she walked into that party on Long Island, where they met, she just knocked him over, he had never seen anyone more beautiful. I think of Doren being loved and appreciated by a man and it makes me feel good, makes me think of her in yet another way.

I keep touching her hands, her soft skin, thinking of how I'll never be able to touch her again. I concentrate on how her hand feels in my hand. I look so often at her hands, examining them, memorizing them. The image of Doren's hands is strong for me. They are so similar to mine. But more delicate. They have always been more delicate.

I will miss Doren's arms around me, the feeling of her lips on my cheek.

She knows what is happening to her. She looked at me from her hospital bed the other day with an expression of horror, pain, and sadness. That look told me she knows. I wish that pain I saw on her face did not exist for her. She's suffering with the illness and also the knowledge of it. I just keep holding her hand, touching her, massaging away the frown between her eyebrows. I pray that at least there is something peaceful in her sleep. And in my loving her.

I was screaming at nurses who insisted I leave the room while they changed Doren's sheets or turned her over. I wanted them to leave her alone. Every time she was moved, she would moan in pain. Doren had only weeks to live and the nurses were shifting her around constantly, disturbing her peace, intent on preventing bedsores.

Doren grew less and less coherent. When I entered the hospital room, I entered Doren's world. Reality became her thoughts, her few words, her needs. There were others who came to be with Doren. Isshin, and the woman he was soon to marry, Elizabeth, sat quietly with me around Doren's bed. Isshin and Doren had developed a close friendship before she became ill, and Doren and Elizabeth had grown fond of each other as well. We were connected during those silent hours inside of Doren's breathing, inside of her life.

Where are you? everywhere your words are fresh,
green leaves on my bed   I gather and spread them all

day long   you are luminous movement
your body is the corps de ballet   your face rising
like lost dreams   becoming my face

My father sat for long periods in the dark room. I always
seemed to be leaving as he was arriving. There was tension
between my parents and me. Arguments, raised voices, cruel
words. We couldn't find a way to manage each other. My
parents bickered. I was enraged. My mother entered the room,
kept her coat on, left quickly. I was enraged. I wanted to make
her stay. I couldn't tolerate her agony.

There was Rob. He rarely left the room. He watched Doren.
Sketched her.

4 MARCH 1981

Tonight at the hospital, as Doren sleeps, I look through
Rob's large sketchbook. Through all of this, all stages of
Doren's illness, he has been sketching her. When I first
noticed him doing this I thought it morbid, perverse. At
least odd. It made me uncomfortable. I had no desire to
see what he was drawing. Yesterday Rob was sitting in a
chair behind me as I leaned over Doren, listening carefully. . . . "Remember . . . I remember you . . . remember
everything. . . ." Rob was witness to this moment. I asked
to see his book. I started from the first page and slowly
allowed every page to enter. The drawings were beautiful.
They were emotionally true. So much emotion expressed
in gestures. My father's particular slouch, the way he nods
off in the chair, the bend of his back, his rounded shoulders. His pain. And Doren. The plea, the quiet, the confusion, the pain, the peace. These drawings are not
unpleasant at all, they are not a record of death. They are
a record of life. I agree with Rob. Doren is beautiful even
now. In fact, her beauty now is so clear, so pure, so vivid.
Uninterrupted.

It becomes harder and harder to leave her. Tonight, as I
was getting ready to leave, I didn't wake her up to say
goodnight, see you tomorrow. I did not want to disturb
the peace in her deep sleeping. Lightly, I kissed her cheek
that was turned to me. Her high cheekbone.

your smiling face
unique and separate from me
adheres to some deeper

tissue and cannot be shaken
loose

13 MARCH 1981

Listening to Doren breathe. There will be a moment when this breathing will stop. When the blood in her veins will stop. When cells will stop multiplying. Doren's soft skin, delicate hands. I will no longer be able to touch her. Her voice. What will it be like to never hear her voice again? I have been watching my sister die.

So afraid of that last breath. She hiccoughed three times tonight. Rob and I, touching her hand and arm, looked up at her, at each other, startled, terrified. Flood of adrenaline through our bodies. It felt as if my breathing would also stop. . . .

Just read Robert Frost's *Birches* again for the first time in a decade and I am flooded with memories. Especially when I remembered my good friend Dorie, at Trebor, reciting it by memory on top of a White Mountain and then shouting, "I am a swinger of birches!" as she swung from a tall and scary (to me) birch. . . .

. . . I don't want her to die in pain. Her sleeping seems peaceful, although the sound of her breathing is raw and deep. . . .

There is no word to describe how I feel inside (writing is so ineffective when you can't think) and here comes my mother and I must do French because I have to get a good mark so I can get into a good college where I can be happy and meet the man of my dreams and, after a fulfilling career, settle down and be happy and at peace and die without pain because I will be immortal and HAPPY. . . .

. . . When my sister is awake, her suffering and anguish cut through everything else existing in the world. . . .

Howdy Doody, Rootie Kazootie
Magic Cottage, Ding Dong School

Perry Como, Captain Video
Winky Dink and Twilight Zone

Kate Smith, Kukla, Fran and Ollie
Sea Hunt and American Bandstand

Ed Sullivan, The Merry Milkman
Dinah Shore and so much more. . . .

While some kids learned from Seuss and Grimms
I sang the holy TV hymns

Davy, Davy Crockett, King of the Wild Frontier . . .

   . . . Isshin and Liz arrived. At first I feel this an intrusion, but only briefly. We are all here for Doren. The energy in this room is expansive. . . .

. . . So Meg and Cathy will visit tonight. I said to Cathy on the
telephone, "I love my life now." I love my life now. I am with
my loved ones again. . . .

   . . . Breathing. My breathing was just now synchronized
with Doren's. . . .

I will tell you how it is here.
Fragrant. Fresh split oak and
jasmine blossoms, evergreen and
cedar, hickory smoke and basil
and dill and hay. . . .

I will tell you how it is here.
Vast. 360° of pink
and blue sky, hundreds of acres
of forest and fields, and only
us

   . . . I must let go of Doren.

Crows and crickets, horses and
cats, chainsaw and axe . . .

Symphonic. I will tell you how it is here. . . .

I have run away with everything that smells like your soft skin. Wearing your cotton sweaters, I bring you in with soft touches of familiarity. Do you miss me where you are? Do you call me in when the visions of all of us throb away from your light into our own colors? I suspect we are closer even than before, but in the ways we used to laugh, I'm caught up now in the sound of it and still hopeful. Loose clothes and dark hair touching your pale neck. I thrash in my wild sleep the cottonwood, the honeysuckle, the lady fern, growing up around our old hiding places, without you.

I seem to be searching around *inside* the sky, as if it were possible for something to turn up there, like the flesh of my life, or perhaps yours, which then would lead me into mine again. The slate-gray songs. They pick themselves up and fly through my sleep, like winter.

THE LAKES HAVE BEEN COMING DOWN FROM THE
MOUNTAINS FOR A LONG TIME

It's already happened, something that occurred
before now
someone's foot (my foot) slipping into
the yielding forest floor (there was only rock
on the north side of the mountain, where I have come
    from)
ankle-deep in fresh growth, ferns bending at my waist
and then the other foot slipping
in too

it is harder this way, climbing down
to a place where I imagine
(all that I had to do, living close
to the jagged peak, was imagine)
lily pads floating around my bare legs
rainwater; warm pools settled into the valley

How impossible to confuse fatigue with desire
but it has only been one year
out of hiding
(timber line; ice water)
and every time I put my ear to the ground
I hear the progress
of your descent on another trail
the long silences during the day
the night struggles

We echo into the same earth

the lakes
have been coming down from the mountains
for a long time

*T*here were the phone calls that had to be made. I volunteered to make them. "I'm sorry to have to tell you this, but Doren died yesterday. We're having a service on Wednesday. . . ." One call after the other, going through Doren's little black phone book, entering what was her world, making contact with her current and past friends. "I don't know whether you know this or not, but Doren had been ill with cancer. . . ."

Who would she want me to call? Who were the names in her book I didn't recognize? Would they want to know? How well did they know Doren? What piece of Doren's life is this that I know nothing about?

On the day of Doren's service, before reading my poem *The Lakes Have Been Coming Down from the Mountains for a Long Time*, and a poem Doren had written before she died, I spoke about Doren and the cornucopia of her writing I had found. After the service, when everyone returned to Mother and George's house, people came up to me and told me how brave it was for me to get up and speak, how amazing I was, how my strength helped them. "I never could have done what you did," they all said. Was I supposed to say thank you? I said nothing. I stared at everyone blankly. Puzzled. What were they praising me for? How could I *not* talk about Doren at her service? She was there. I was making a connection with my sister, I was talking to *her*.

It has been ten days. This is only the beginning of missing Doren. The impulse, inside of so many moments, is to share with her. This deep, profound impulse as natural as any of my other senses.

Doren. I just want to write her name, say her name, think her name, call her name. She is gone. Doren has died. But she is still here, inside of me, talking to me, laughing with me, strong and present. Her voice coming into my dreams.

22 March 1981. A Sunday. We hated Sundays. When we were children the worst family arguments would occur on Sunday. Ten fifty-four P.M. Jeffrey's arrival back at his house, where I have been waiting for him, four minutes before Doren dies. I am where I need to be; my father is where he needs to be, with his niece, Jackie, who has come from Ohio to be with him; my mother is where she needs to be, with George and his sister, Claire. Doren knew this. She was with us all at that moment. Peaceful, releasing herself into another world. Into the light. I felt her free. I felt myself confined.

I keep imagining the moment of Doren's passing. The moment life swept out of her body. The final collapse of her physical presence. The letting go. The release. The final acceptance. Rob was holding her, her head on his shoulder, he was helping the nurse turn Doren. When Rob described the moment to me, he only cried. There is no description. There is only my image, again and again.

Holding Doren. Won't I always be holding Doren?

I will never know her aging. As I grow older she will still be thirty-three. Soon there will no longer be four years between us. I will be older than my older sister. Nature has slipped. A terrible error. The natural order of the physical world has changed. An awkward, devastating shift.

Is it possible you begin to understand love only after someone you love has died?

We went to Doren's apartment the day after she died with boxes, newspapers, twine. Packing up everything that belonged to her was a gruesome task. Dismantling her carefully put-together home. I had the bedroom to take apart—the pastel angora sweaters sweet with Doren's perfume, the winter dresses that had not been stored for spring, the silk scarves, the bookshelf filled with loose-leaf journals. George had the living room—all those books, Doren's bulletin board, her desk, her papers, her unfinished novel. My mother had the kitchen —the Arabia dishes that were a wedding gift to Doren and

Andrew, the French and Italian tinted glassware, countless wooden utensils, sturdy silverware. Claire was helping my mother in the kitchen. My father hadn't come. It wouldn't have been wise for my mother and father to be together now—their emotions were frayed and bristling and there was too much chance for a clash.

Mother came into the bedroom. She saw me sitting on the floor by the bed, holding one of Doren's journals in my lap. I had glanced inside, then closed it quickly. I felt like the young teenager again, peeking at Doren's journal behind her back. "I have to tell you something," Mother said. I looked at her face, but not exactly at her eyes. (Was it years before we were able to look into each other's eyes again? Was I afraid I would find Doren in hers, was she afraid she'd find Doren in mine?) "George went to identify Doren's body today." He had offered to do this. He was protecting my mother, perhaps my father too. George had been taking care of all of us. Who, I wondered, was taking care of George? I put down the journal, found him in the living room, put my arms around him. "Thank you," I said. I could tell he was crying and didn't want me to know. I wondered how long he would have to be my mother's protector, how long he would have to go unprotected. George was suffering the loss of Doren as well.

It is late April and I'm just getting around to my taxes. My accountant wonders how I can be bothering with taxes now, given the fact that my sister has just died. Another one wondering how I, or anyone else who experiences tragedy, can function.

I have been thinking about this business of "functioning." I know that I am functioning. That is not really a mystery to me. I think I am also, in some important ways, thriving. Sometimes there are glimmers of richness in my life.

Damp, fresh summer air today. The caulking is off all windows, and the windows are open. This morning I transferred a message that Doren had left on my phone machine months ago onto my tape recorder. A permanent record of her voice. When I imagine her voice, which I do all the time, it causes me great pain. When I actually hear it on tape, it is so natural to listen to.

So much Doren. Dreams most every night bring me into a disturbing morning. What is not possible—Doren's non-existence—is what is real. And not real. Doren. Even the name is so much the person. I miss saying her name, and when I use it talking to a friend, I am happy to be able to say the name. But no more calling to her in another room, "Dor-en!" Or calling her on the phone, "Dor?" Or hearing her say, "Cath?"

In so many dreams Doren dies over and over again. The nightmare stretches into endless dark shapes. Does one keep trying to get death right? To bring it into life in some recognizable shape so that it will become less frightening? Does one try to make death a companion? If Doren is my sister, then isn't death my sister as well? Death suddenly became something that belonged to Doren. It was something inside her body, not a nameless external force. I watched death become visible as a part of my sister's life. But isn't death always there? We just don't see it. We carry, inside of us, the dark companion.

There was the "vacation" in Key Biscayne with Mother and George just weeks after Doren's death. The tension between all of us was unbearable. Mother and George fought. Mother thought they would separate. I knew this was crazy. I knew we were all out of control.

Portuguese man-of-war in the ocean. Warning signs. Warning signs. When I was eight years old, playing the right hand of Heart and Soul on the piano, Doren playing the left hand, I didn't know she was going to die. I didn't know the pain I would have to watch her endure. I didn't know that our last coupling would be when I was twenty-nine and she was thirty-three.

I don't even feel alone right now. I don't feel. A hand puppet in the attic trunk. Resigned, having no other choice.

I can't link anything about my physical presence, and the physical world, with Doren's physical absence.

I said to a friend the other early evening, sipping a Bloody Mary on Columbus Avenue, that I am still walking around as someone's sister. You *are* one, my friend says. But I'm not. Not anymore. My identity has been altered. The unusually warm spring afternoon that day was marked. It was marked with missing Doren.

A decision had been made to bury Doren's ashes on Candice's farm. It had been Doren's place, her place of peace.

Candice was her closest friend, and Candice's mother and husband also loved Doren. My mother was uneasy with the decision. Virginia was not a place she would be able to get to very often, and she wanted a place where, she explained, she could go and be with Doren. Her first choice was her own property in East Hampton, but I knew this wouldn't sit well with my father since he would never feel comfortable visiting there. I was in the middle and without my sister as ally. I was furious with Doren for not being there to help me manage our parents. Now, they were *my* parents. All this conflict, mixed with loss, postponed the burying of the ashes for six months. My father was outraged. He had wanted to do it immediately. He threatened to go without us. To take the ashes and run. This didn't happen.

My defenses were as liquid as rain. There was sadness. Resentment. Invasive loneliness. My cat's death followed just weeks after Doren's. The vet called me to come in. The cat was still alive, wrapped in a towel, lying motionless on a metal table. I walked into that room, heard the breathing. The same breathing. The presence of death was unmistakable.

> This sense of being alone, this bleakness, hopelessness, absence of joy. I walk around in a cocoon, quietly, gentle steps. Inside of the hazy quiet, the thought: *Something terrible has happened, everything from here on is tenuous, perishable.*
>
> Mother says she can't believe, when she's walking down the street, that that whole big person isn't here anymore. That whole big person. Vanished.
>
> I walk in the door expecting my cat to be inside. I walk in the door. Expecting.
>
> The cliff's edge, the wind at my back; leaning.

I searched for people who would allow me my grief. I began to move away from those who would not. While Doren was dying, our relationship and my need to be with her took precedence over everything else. After Doren died, other needs began to matter again. Having people around me I could trust and count on mattered.

One of the people I could rely on for comfort, understanding, and something akin to spiritual guidance was a woman who, many years earlier, had been Doren's bunk-mate at our camp and Doren's close friend. The similarities between them were numerous, including their names—Doren and Dorien.

They were also both writers. Dorien, or Dorie, did not become a close friend of mine until just a year or so before Doren had become ill. She had reconnected with Doren and me not long after the sudden death of her brother. Dorie was now living in California, and through letters, phone calls, and her visits to see her parents in New York, Dorie and I developed a bond.

Dorie and her brother were close siblings, and when she told me her brother had died I couldn't help but think of Doren and me. This was before Doren had become ill. Dorie's brother had died on Doren's birthday. He had been the first boy Doren had developed a crush on when she was a young teenager. I never expected Dorie and I would, in the near future, share the experience of the death of a sibling. We would develop an intimacy through the sharing of grief and through the rebuilding of our lives. The fact that we would become siblings ourselves, not by blood but through this experience, would simultaneously strengthen and disrupt our relationship.

My thirtieth birthday was looming large before me in June, just a little over two months after Doren died. I kept seeing the large numbers in front of my face, they shone on and off like neon—3 0 3 0 3 0 3 0. The numbers were telling me to *do* something, *change* something, take *ACTION*.

It was a clean sweep, a swift changing of gears. I left Jeffrey for the final time, I left my therapist, I decided it was time to take my acting seriously and I began to go out on auditions. I was *busy*, busier than I had ever been in my life. There was no time to ponder, there was only time to *DO*. My vision of time had altered radically, and I had to move *FAST*. I was hurtling through space at inhuman speeds. I kept trying to get out of the way of my pain, and I kept stumbling into it.

> 8 June 1981. Thirty. Last night I put Doren's rings on my fingers. The two she wore to the end.
>
> Little blue antique glass Doren bought me, next to this typewriter (Doren's), with red wine in it. This is a hard birthday. So incredibly hard.
>
> Thirty.
>
> Gene says, "Strut your stuff, Cathy, get out there and strut your stuff."
>
> A little drunk now. Nervous. Hopeful.

During that summer a job possibility came my way. A movie producer was looking for someone to be his assistant and I was being considered for the job. There were extensive interviews in New York and then an all-expenses-paid trip to Los Angeles in August. The activity was a blessing. It was as if a deus ex machina had scooped me up out of my misery and deposited me into a brighter world. The people I met did not know about Doren's death. Relief.

A chauffeur and limousine met me at the airport and took me to my hotel suite. Champagne awaited me, and the keys to a rented car. I was aware of how bizarre this all was. My sister had just died, I was mourning, and there I was sipping champagne while taking a bath.

After my stint in Los Angeles was completed, I decided to visit Dorie in Berkeley. We didn't talk about grief. I didn't want to. I thought, perhaps, my grief was over. After all, hadn't I been mourning since the time Doren first had cancer? As far as I wanted to know, I had already paid my dues regarding grief. Dorie was watching me closely. She knew what I was up against, she knew I was protecting myself by holding the virulent sorrow at bay. Had she told me this then, I would have insisted I was just fine.

On the deck at Dorie's house, a late August day. The sun is on me. Mountains across the way. I want to live here. I'm peaceful in California. The tension is gone. My body is grateful.

Dorie returns from Yosemite. When I come back from running she is sitting on the front steps in a bathrobe and her hair in a towel. Her friend and neighbor, Bettina, is watering flowers on the front lawn. The two large dogs are on the porch.

Twin Peaks. Golden Gate to the left, shelf of fog coming in from the ocean into the bay toward Berkeley. The mountains, sun setting, the houses on the hills, like Hydra or Florence, the bay bridge to the left in the distance, ships. Clear dusk. Baker Beach. Golden Gate close by, lit up. I drive up the mountain. Exhausted from the physical beauty of this place. I feel like I can't take any more beauty in.

21 September 1981. In the air, on the way to Washington, D.C. To Virginia. To bury Doren's ashes. Ashes that were once my sister's body. I want to hurl curses at whoever, whatever, was responsible for her death. Flashes of rage. What remains of her physical presence is tucked into George's bag. Ashes. Bits of bone. Doren's bones.

Mother, George, Claire, and I. This all so strange. We're walking around with Doren's ashes and talking to each other like normal people. I want to scream until I can't scream any more. I'm quiet. Sitting in the back of the plane, away from the others, quiet. I'm acting quiet, I don't feel quiet.

Sitting at the gate waiting to board the plane, I put my hand over George's bag. Protective. Part of my sister is in there. Walking to the gate, I thought, "Doren, we're coming." I know she's going to be there today. She's been waiting for us to come to the farm. I actually feel like I'm going to be visiting Doren today. She thought my first time at the farm would be with her. Maybe she was right.

The site is the promontory. We plant a pink dogwood tree next to the place on the hill where we bury the ashes. Inside the box Rob made (he and my father chose not to come for this ceremony), there are two compartments. One is for the ashes, one is for other things we put in. I choose the tiny gold wishbone charm, with a pearl on one tip, that Doren and I wore when we were children (we had matching charms); rubbings of balsam pine, our favorite smell because it reminded us of Trebor and Maine; and my poem, Doren's favorite—*The Lakes Have Been Coming Down from the Mountains for a Long Time*—the last of my writing she ever read. Candice adds basil leaves from her garden —she had always given Doren basil leaves to take home with her.

I read my poem. Unlike reading it at the service for Doren six months before, this time I can barely get through it. We plant the tree. We each put dirt on the box. I hear water moving below; the brook. This is a place Doren would love, I think, especially because it is in the shade. She hated the sun to burn her skin. I would always be in the direct line of the sun, Doren would be sitting under a tree.

We walk away in silence. I don't return to New York with my family. I am going to Maine, to meet a friend there. My plane is delayed for hours. There are storms. Waiting at the gate, I eat candy. One tooth breaks in half. It figures, I think.

She comes to me out of hiding. After her death, she speaks to me in my dreams in a voice I recognize. When this occurs I know the dream is no longer a dream. It is a suspension of time. I have even called Doren out of hiding when I have needed her. She comes to me as she did while playing hide and seek, at the moment when my bewilderment as to her whereabouts was about to turn into a deeper distress. Sometimes before falling off to sleep I plead gently, "Doren, Doren, tonight I need to hear your voice, I need to feel you here with me." I have held back pain with my own arms wrapped around my body as if they were my sister's arms. Sometime during the night I feel Doren's arms take the place of mine.

THE PROMONTORY

Rubbings of balsam and basil
and the tiny gold wishbone, the pearl
move further down.

And it is your voice
folding into the supple ground
into a trail of months, catching up
with the intimate songs we sent
spinning in lakewater to compensate
somehow for your pain.

You still attend to me
and I have been holding you
close to my moods, like reassurance
still unaware of world news
as if you might still come around again
in your high heels and pearl necklace
with information and fun plans for the day.

We said, "We look alike except
for our mouths." It isn't exactly true

that the dead separate from obvious places.
Your expressions coming up on my face.
Stray animals appearing in the glass
keeping warm.

*T*here were months of rage. It became my protection. Put away hurt, put away sadness, put away loss. I walked my way through every aspect and nuance of my rage, saw it, felt it, released myself into the whirlpool. The only way to let it go was to allow it its power. There was a calmer place through the bottom of the whirlpool. Doren, at the end of her life, called rage a poison—poison to the life of the spirit, poison to the life of the body. She taught herself how to let the rage go. Then she taught me.

The cartons stuffed with Doren's belongings were stored in my mother's apartment. They were piled into the closet that once was Doren's, in the room that was once our bedroom. At first, I wanted none of Doren's things. There was harm in objects. Grief settled into her clothes, her dishes, her books, her records. I didn't want what belonged to Doren. I didn't want her pictures.

My mother felt differently. She placed a few articles of Doren's clothing in her drawer. They carried the scent of Doren's perfume. Mother held them up to her face, breathed in deeply for comfort, for Doren's life. And there were the pictures. She held them to her lips, kissed her child.

My father was concerned about Doren's plants. He wanted to know where they were, who was taking care of them. Mother had taken a few, I had taken one. I could handle Doren's plant. It was a living thing. My father didn't ask for anything from the cartons. He wanted only the pictures. Doren at camp, on visiting day, white shorts, white blouse, white pixie band, looking away from the camera. Doren, twenty, a formal portrait, hair pulled back, black liner on her eyelids, an imperceptible smile. Doren and I at the piano. Children's fingers.

George kept watch over my mother. I watched him watching her intently. She could no longer press Doren to her body, all that was left to her was grief, so she held it close as she would her child. George circled around his wife's grief, trying either to coax her away from its hold or be admitted in. Mother was holding Doren now, her daughter was swaddled in stark white grief, and she would allow no one to share her burden. George watched her and could do little.

We all retreated from each other. Rob disappeared back into

his life. We gave him Doren's furniture to take with him. I stayed away from my parents. My mother and father were no longer speaking. They had conceived and raised a daughter together, who had died, and they would never share their grief over that death. Months went by. I was putting all my energy into managing life, instigating changes, moving into my future as fast as I could, as fast as I could get away from Doren's death.

Which decision came first—to begin acting professionally or to begin to lift the lids of the cartons? I began to go to auditions: I was dressed in Doren's clothes. I took on her black sweaters, her suede high-heeled shoes, her pearls, her sophistication. Friends commented. "I love your sweater," they'd say. "Doren's," I'd say. And still do. "Thanks," I say, "it's Doren's." If I don't say this, I feel I am cheating.

"You belong on a stage," Doren had said. Exactly one year after Doren died, I was cast in my first show. Now I was on a stage, and I would begin to write again as well. My isolation was less consuming, less threatening. I could submit to solitude and also be a part of the world. Doren was with me. I could feel her touch. Every few months I would continue the quiet and slow search through the cartons. Slowly, I brought Doren home with me.

20 June 1982. Will I go on counting this way, year after year? Today Doren would have been thirty-five. Next year —thirty-six. And so on. Always four years older than I. As if there were days still to be counted in her life. As if she were still being filled with years. As if she were still in relationship to this side of time.

Goddamn it, I miss her. And I want to keep counting.

I returned to California during the summer of 1982. First I visited Dorie in Berkeley. Immediately after I arrived at her house, the poems began. They were emerging, one after the other, and they were all about Doren. I stayed awake through the night. I wrote, and I wrote, and I wrote. Dorie read the poems. She held me. "Cathy," she said, "you have found your voice. You have found your voice about your sister."

24 August 1982. Here's the story—There is an orange tree outside the bathroom window. I can see the same orange tree through the kitchen window when I am sitting at the table eating breakfast. There are two huge picture

windows in the main room and when I am sitting here at the desk I am looking out at the Berkeley hills. It is so nourishing here I feel like I'm going to burst. The house is so bright it is as if the sun has moved inside with me.

The sun setting over the ocean here is an extraordinary event. Witnessing the meeting of these two great forces. And the sky, turning soft blues and pinks, in compliance. Letting go.

Dorie introduces me to a man who cooks me a dinner of whole trout with browned, sautéed sliced almonds over the length of the fish, and rice with tomatoes, mushrooms, onions, and other necessary things. The almond-colored wine tastes like champagne. The seduction is quiet, sweet, and welcome. The memory of this rhythm comes tumbling back to me, a huge tumbleweed, feather-light, rolling into town at a silent, breakneck speed, from out of the desert and the dry wind, full of color, all the things it has picked up on its journey that are close to the earth, and suddenly I think that what was lost to me is here again, with me, present.

In Los Angeles I made the necessary professional appointments in my pursuit of acting work. The most important appointment, however, was not because of what it brought me professionally but because of what it brought me personally. At that time Peter Bogdanovich was immersed in writing his book—*The Killing of the Unicorn*—about Dorothy Stratten and her tragic death. He talked to me about Dorothy. I talked to him about Doren. There were so few places safe enough for grief. Peter understood. I sat in his sun-drenched living room as he spoke softly about the calico cat that had sauntered into his house nine months after Dorothy was murdered. He had noticed an unusual marking on the cat's face. Dorothy had once given Peter a greeting card with a photograph of a calico kitten—the marking on the face in the photograph, and the marking on the face of the cat that stood in Peter's living room, were identical. The cat that suddenly appeared never left. I, too, had experienced events we could find no other word for but "mystical." We were not swapping stories of loss and grief, but rather were celebrating the spirits of the women we had loved most in the world. Were we finding ways for these women to stay with us? Were these women letting us know they would always stay?

The poems continued after I returned to New York. They

were my morning ritual for a year. Arising early morning, propping up my pillows, lighting a candle by the bed, sipping a large mug of coffee, I would write.

THE FIRST YEAR

Tell the farmer his chickens
are creeping around before sunup
and the plaid flannel shirt
on the scarecrow has not brought order
to the unseen chaos of the corn

I've forgotten what it is that survives—
the boulder above the ocean
the gray cellar
the distance between one city and another

if I've wept it's because
the vegetation around placid lakewater
is tangled up with my ankles
and if I grieve
it is from peeling layers of mica
off the side of a mountain

learn to take the sound
of your favorite screen door
out of your dreams
and the easy height of the red barn
may tell you another story

8 October 1982. Jeffrey and I happen upon each other yesterday. The first thing I notice is his height. I am struck by it. This tallness I did not remember, though certainly I remembered he was tall. Later, when feelings about Doren come careening back to me, I wonder whether his height was such a surprise because, perhaps unconsciously, I shrunk him down to Doren's size, fit him into Doren's body. Last night I ask Doren to come to me in my sleep. She does. She presses her body to mine. We are standing. We hold each other. She holds me all night, reminding me of her presence.

After Doren died, mail continued to arrive for her. It was being forwarded to my mother's address. At first every week an envelope would arrive with Doren's name on it. Then there would be a lapse. Then her name would appear again, lying on the doormat with the rest of the day's mail. Mother would call and, in a voice barely audible, would tell me something had arrived, again, for Doren. It was disturbing. A small detail of death.

I was over at Mother and George's apartment on a Saturday when they were out of town. It was only when my mother wasn't home that I would go through the cartons. If she was there, she would appear in the room, watch me try on Doren's clothes. I'd notice her tears. She wouldn't leave, though, and I wouldn't ask her to. On this particular Saturday a letter came for Doren. This hadn't occurred in many months.

It was an aerogram from England. Doren had had a friend who lived in London. Oh my God, I thought, she doesn't know Doren died. Had I missed her name in Doren's phone book? I opened the letter. She was puzzled that she had not heard from Doren in so long. There was no mention of Doren's illness. Had Doren never told her about the cancer?

I didn't want to burden my mother. I began to think about how and what I was going to write to Doren's friend. I've never composed that letter. For years I have been waiting for an idea to come to me, a way in which I can deflate the information.

Then there was Rubie, a woman who lived with our family when Doren and I were children. She didn't know either. Rubie had taken care of us when our parents were away over extended periods of time. Doren and I became attached to her, and as our parents' marriage grew more and more tumultuous, we relied on Rubie for stability and constant attention. She gave us both.

Every Christmas, and on our birthdays, Doren and I would receive a card from Rubie. Even after twenty years had passed since she had seen us, we still heard from her. The Christmas after Doren died, I heard from Rubie. She asked in her note if I would please send her Doren's address, she had misplaced it. I didn't respond. The following Christmas she made the same request. I was still stumped. How could I tell her?

This year, when another card from Rubie arrived, I did not stuff it away in a file. I couldn't hide anymore from the dreaded, written words—My sister died.

I wrote to Rubie and I told her about Doren.

There have also been the phone calls. Doren's old friends who heard of her death long after it occurred. One call in particular was more disturbing than the others. It was from Jamie.

He and Doren had known each other as teenagers and briefly as adults while Doren was still married to Andrew. I was startled to hear from Jamie and surprised even more when he began to talk, nonstop, about how shocked he was, how upset, how he had heard the news, how he had really *known* Doren. He did not pause to ask how I was. When I tried to interject, he cut me off. When he completed his monologue, he asked me for every detail about what had happened to Doren. He didn't merely inquire—he demanded. He didn't care how his questions might have affected me. He seemed to care only about soothing himself.

Jamie wanted to arrange a time when we could meet and talk. I rattled off my busy schedule and told him this really wasn't a very good time for me. He accused me of hedging. He thought I owed him something. "You're trying to avoid me," he scolded. I would have said, "Yes, that's true," but I didn't want to make any personal confessions to him. Jamie grew more and more angry—and adamant. He continued to press me, and when he didn't get what he wanted he declared that he would be sure to call back and try again.

I knew that what Jamie wanted was not to see me at all. The person he wanted to see was Doren. He wanted me to *be* Doren. He was as surprised at being turned down by me as he would have been had it been Doren. He wanted to fill the loss of Doren with me as the substitute.

I was relieved that I never heard from him again.

22 March 1983. It is Doren I want to talk to, Doren's absence that surrounded the house in Merrick this past Sunday. I drove out there. Searching. The car stalled on our old block. I have no business here anymore, I thought. I'm never coming back.

"The wind took me away." Why didn't he take me too? "Because he only likes me."

This missing begins to have a life of its own, flouncing about like an injured fish, its belly touching down here and there on the bottom of the ocean. Sea plants flex their wisdom and I have entertained notions, some more violent than others. The violence is held at bay by the missing.

My dreams are diligent. Like a battery of exams, on one subject only, they go straight through. Meanwhile, taking advantage of the situation, the candle leaps right into the radiator. In the morning, I have to look for it. There it is, the wick elongated and exposed, the warm wax melted down, curved into an obvious phallic shape. There is a motor running in the next room, but I can't find the source. Then I do. Under its gray plastic cover, the typewriter had turned itself on. Your old typewriter. Tearing the cover off, I stare at the phenomenon. That familiar hum, going on during the night without me. Abruptly, I flick the switch to Off. Then to On again, then Off, place both hands on the casing; a benediction. The heat is startling. Confirming. Let's just say I had a visitor last night. I call out to your spirit. Asking the usual questions.

A FORM OF GREETING

The slim fire moving up stalks
is a form of greeting
active, each day comes careening forth
and we try to hold what we can put our arms around

your best friend is encouraging
she helps you move your couch to another part of the
    room
you remember her hair when it was longer
and suddenly you are stronger than anything as
    arrogant
as separation

our feet flat on the ground becomes a kind of joke
even solid objects have their limits;   a rim

in the West, the sky and the ocean are in agreement
the sky lets go of the sun, the ocean takes it

sailcloth gives in the wind
even the billowing light
will move out into silence

and yet we take whatever it is we have been saving
in darkness, out

I was acting, I was writing, I was finding new friendships, I was looking my best. Everyone was proud of me.

Something was missing. It was joy. If I went down deep into
either elation or sorrow, I was sure to find Doren. I was unwilling to bring my feelings about her absence to life. How
could I experience joy if Doren would never be there again to
share it with me.

The healing began with a move toward gentleness. Finally, I
allowed a nurturing man into my life. I found the comfort
Doren's death had taken away. Rod helped me find my way
back to Doren's life. I would discover her life, and mine, apart
from death.

The kinship I had with Rod I had known before. I had lost it
when my sister died. As some people search for their mother
or their father in a mate, I was searching for my sister.

Rod had to move to Denver for a year, and he left during the
summer of '83. What I felt that summer was a strong desire to
leave New York. I wanted to go somewhere where I could feel
myself separate from the parts of my life I felt were holding me
fast to my childhood. My own home held too much acute
memory, and my relationships did as well.

It had been two years since Doren had died, and for the first
time since then I remembered my last words to her. She was
in a coma. It was the last time I would ever see her. No one
was in the room but me. I made her a promise. "Doren," I
whispered, "your writing will be published. I will make sure
of that."

I planned to go to California in August, and I planned to
take Doren's journals with me. I hadn't read them yet. Now
I was ready to. In Los Angeles, I could also pursue acting
work.

August 31, 1983. Moving day. A house in Los Angeles that I
had sublet for a few months was waiting for me. I was all
packed. Cartons had already been shipped out. They included
Doren's journals. I had, the night before, celebrated with all
my friends at a restaurant in Little Italy. Now I was off. For the

first time since before my sister had become ill, I was feeling joy. That joy included Doren. I felt confident—and I felt strong enough to take Doren with me.

On the morning of August 31, I went for my last run in Central Park. It looked more beautiful to me than ever. I would miss running here. It was 9 A.M. There was a morning mist. It was peaceful.

My world, my joy, my peace was shattered within minutes. That morning, as I was finishing my usual four-mile run, I was raped.

I also survived.

Survival. Had I ever been closer to Doren than in those moments when I almost lost my own life? Doren did not survive the violence of her disease, but my sister was never a victim. She was a survivor. When death approached, Doren held on to her life. While she was alive darkness wouldn't claim her. The pulse of her life was vibrant color. Here was the core of Doren's legacy to me. I would refuse the persona of victim. I would retrieve the vibrant colors. I would be a survivor.

A year later, after treatment that was crucial to my healing, I would become a volunteer counselor for rape survivors. I had learned, in a group with other women who had survived rape, that healing was possible. I wanted to share that knowledge and encourage that capacity in others. I would remember the feelings Doren described when she taught retarded adults and children. I thought Doren had the ability to give in a way that I did not. I used to wonder why she would want, voluntarily, to expose herself to the sorrow and difficulties of strangers. I wondered how, exactly, the joy arose out of sorrow. I would find another part of my sister that was also part of me.

Within a week of the rape I flew to California, then promptly transported myself and the cartons with all those journals to a safe place. That place was with Rod, in Denver. The rage I had felt during my sister's illness and after her death erupted with a vengeance. I couldn't grieve for myself without grieving for Doren. The world was without grace, and I matched its lumbering spirit with my own. Rod held me and, in so doing, he held me to the world.

As Doren had. They were connected.

22 March 1984. Here we are again, Doren. Your picture, a candle, my typewriter. The third anniversary of your death. I think we're still together, but I feel like I'm losing track of the ways we're together now.

It's different. There's distance from the acute pain.

The pink petals of the dogwood tree on the site where Doren's ashes are buried. Doren's ashes under the ground, my poem, balsam, a gold wishbone. A third spring is now approaching. Only the third. She has missed only two. So short a time. So long a time to miss her.

I have been learning this lesson: When I let go there is lightness, vulnerability, joy. I learned this by watching how much Doren chose to live before she died.

It is not death that teaches us lessons. It is the way we choose to be in the light, or darkness, of any given fate.

My sister did not die in order for me to come to life. I chose to live after her death.

For three years after my sister's death, my relationship to her was mostly through pain. When the pain lessened I needed to discover in what other ways we could be together. Pain had been the vehicle keeping me with my sister. I knew there had to be a way for us to be together that was more life-enhancing, but it wasn't clear to me what it was.

I used to think losing the pain meant losing Doren. I began to see that it meant I was giving Doren back to herself. Making myself whole, I was allowing Doren her own identity again.

Doren died, and I take on new parts of her. I take on new beauty so that Doren's beauty is not lost. In finding my own strength, I am making room for Doren's strength to enter. Within my freedom, Doren, too, is free.

Remember . . . remember . . . I remember you, I remember you. . . .

These pictures surround me, accompany me. Doren and I as children. As adults. Separately. Together. Always touching. The sisterhood continues. It continues to bring sustenance.

THE LEGACY

No council is kept here
but deep in the woods
where things have overgrown
at protective angles
there is a wide circle of rocks
all the same, all flat, all low to the ground

it is the only wisdom
the molding of iron into potbellied stoves
is less poignant

civilization that has taught our hands
to close around useful things
employed the principle of coming up out of water:
the hand grasps anything resembling shore
a piece of driftwood, a protrusion on the side of a boat

in between the small rocks
there is also the legacy of the flutes

there are trees in the spaces
where our fingers should go

I drove across the country from Denver to New York. I was returning. I sang my heart out, cried, laughed— with the steady rhythm of road, barns, farmland, cows, road, barns, flatland, dust storms, I began to remember. Stuffed into the car with me were all my cartons, all the journals.

Before leaving Denver I went to California to act in Peter Bogdanovich's film *Mask*. This led me back to my creative spirit.

I knew Doren was with me.

In June I had a birthday. Thirty-three. The age at which Doren died.

20 June 1984. Doren's birthday. Mine a couple of weeks ago. My parents seem to be better than I am today. I am thirty-three now. Doren, when she had her thirty-third birthday on this day, would not have another one. I am fearing for my life. And somehow fearing for Doren's life, too, imagining, or trying to, how it would be to die at age thirty-three. I start to imagine and then retreat from such thoughts. I reject that darkness, that all-out utter fear.

Dear Cathy—

I have just returned from Russia, and I want to send you this picture right away. It was taken in the town of Suzdal, from a dirt path leading toward the Kremlin. Inside the fortress, on the left, you can see the Cathedral of the Nativity of the Virgin. In the middle distance is the river Kamenka, with three men fishing through a hole they have cut in the ice.

There is an ancient tradition that Russian earth should be brought and placed on the grave of a Russian who has died on foreign soil. And so Mama and I picked up a little soil just at the spot from which I took this picture. I have saved this for Doren, and here is why.

When Doren and I first met in the fall of 1965 at Bryn Mawr, she liked to call me a lumberjack, inspired by her first sight of me. We were both in the public bathroom of the dorm late one night. I was wearing a plaid flannel shirt, leaning over the sink, and stirring my coffee with my thumb. And so the conversation started.

Doren told me all about herself, about you, her parents, and eventually about her Russian grandfather who had once pronounced that a man should have big hands and big feet. Otherwise, he's not to be trusted. Doren also told me that someone, I can't remember who it was, called her a Russian princess. I have always thought of her as one.

I'll save the Russian soil for your next visit, if you like.

Love,
Candice

I wasn't able to move back into my apartment until August. My landlords, a married couple, both of whom are architects, had moved into my home and made it their office. They refused to budge. I was immediately immersed in a legal and highly emotionally charged battle. While I looked for an apartment to sublet I stayed with my mother and George. This was the apartment I had been a child in. Now I welcomed my mother's nurturing. I did not feel endangered by it, I was not regressing into childhood. Mother was so happy to now have the opportunity to attend to me. She understood that I had had to leave in order to return. We could be mother and daughter again. Our lives could touch without one being consumed by the other. Her fear of losing me, her only living child now, was not keeping her from me anymore. We talked about Doren. We hadn't for all the years since her death. We began to listen to each other. We heard each other's sadness.

My father, too, listened. I no longer felt I had to be my sister for my parents. I couldn't compensate for her absence in their lives. My parents saw that I was affirming my own life and that I could still be their daughter.

When I got back into my apartment I had to make it my own. With some of Doren's belongings, and new furniture I bought for myself, I created a place to live and work that was bright, vibrant. I discovered I had lost some friendships during my absence, those that could not incorporate my changes, but I renewed others.

Rod, who was back in New York, was in my life. We were determined that our relationship would not be a casualty of crisis and grief and our own fears of intimacy. I used to wonder how I would ever be able to share my life with someone who had never known Doren. How would he understand? I no longer feel that way. I have no doubt that Rod knows her, and understands.

I am sometimes bursting with dreams that seem very far away. . . .I am at ease with myself, confident, and not afraid . . . we sail out beyond our bodies to a common ground . . . or ocean. . . .

The twenty-second of March 1985. I am accustomed to

mourning on this day. It is the four-year anniversary of Doren's death. Today *Mask* opens around the country. Doren had a hand in this, I think. I hear her saying—You can't be sorrowful on this day. You are in your life now. You must rejoice.

In a few days I will be thirty-four. Thirty-three will have passed. On the last birthday of mine that Doren was alive for, she gave me a card. The cancer was in remission. We didn't know that within a year she would die. And yet it seems as if Doren felt then that perhaps the rest of my birthdays would go on without her.

June 1980. Happy birthday, dearest sister. May the coming years bring you fulfillment, adventure, and joy. You are full of gifts, and I know these gifts will help you find your way.

I love you
Doren

One weekend, while I was in Colorado, I went on a trip offered by Outward Bound, a survival-training school. The snow in the mountains was waist-deep. I walked across ropes raised high off the ground. I inched along wooden beams from one tree to another. I skied cross-country through a blizzard. On the last day, the Outward Bound leaders suggested we take our journals and find a solitary place on the mountain. We were not supposed to return to shelter for two hours.

I couldn't feel my fingers under three pairs of woolen socks I had covered my hands with. I could barely hold the pen I had brought with me. I was consumed with the task of keeping warm. The snow. The cold. My cold fingers. My cold toes. My painful muscles. I fantasized returning to shelter before the two hours were up. There was silence. I listened. . . .

I remember everything, remember everything . . .
I remember you.
I stayed. I began to write. . . .
Our hands on the piano. Playing Chopsticks. Playing Heart and Soul . . .

Doren, this picture is for you.

You could dance.
For years there was
always plenty of music.
You would wonder where it all
came from,
carry small pieces of it to school
and—erasing the
sounds of school—would
lay the music out
one shard at a time
while doodling,
"Mrs.?" "Mrs.???"

Dancing rapidly into the future
out of the here—
even though here
were ballet slippers that looked
alive even when your
feet weren't in them,
and here were
stuffed cabbages on winter nights
and huggable small sister
and hottest showers and
coldest apples
and best, best friends
(who knew all your secrets)—

All of these things,
but most important
the dancing,
sweating
your way out of childhood.
Here was a world that made some
sense. Oh, there was pain—
ooze beneath your blackened
toenails, arms that almost shattered
in the air. Your teacher, too,
would give the cruelest
combinations, but
just move
inches
to the left or to
the right, where it hurt
so much, and sometimes, you were
beautiful.

Doren Arden
December 1980